# Diagnosing and curing IBS with science: a sufferer's guide

by Trevor Klee

# Table of Contents

# Introduction

I went through my own bout with IBS some years ago. It was really frustrating. It seemed to come out of nowhere. I spent a lot of money on a test for SIBO to see if that was the problem, but didn't see any results. Then, it briefly seemed like I was cured, only to randomly become sensitive to gluten for a year.

Dealing with IBS was especially frustrating because of the unhelpful advice from doctors, family, and friends. Doctors would tell me it was all in my head. My family thought I had Crohn's. My friends just would get weirded out by the things I refused to eat, and try to nag me into trying just one muffin/beer/hot wing.

A few years ago, my IBS disappeared as suddenly as it came. Now, I'm mostly ok. But I still remember how frustrating and life-impairing IBS was.

One of the things I really wished I had when I got IBS was an actually helpful guide. When I would Google IBS, I'd get a bunch of blog posts from "reputable" sources that all said the same thing. It was so unhelpful. "Oh, Mayo Clinic, should I avoid foods that trigger my IBS and also try to exercise once a day? Really? Wow, thanks, I'm cured!"

This book is different. It's an actually helpful guide: a scientific way to think about, diagnose, and treat your IBS. Here's how it's laid out.

## The organization of the book

The book is laid out first with a table to make sure you actually have IBS, and not a similar condition. Then it has a table to treat your IBS.

If you have a simpler form of IBS, these two tables might be enough. If you have a more complex form, or a more complex condition, you will need a doctor's help. That's why the next section is how to deal with your doctors, who will likely be your GP and your gastro.

When you're dealing with your doctors (or figuring things out yourself), you should have an idea of how your digestive system actually works. That's why I've put another section here on how your digestive system works, and how it breaks down in the various IBS-related conditions.

At the end of the book, I list all my sources (and there are a lot!) and what I took from them. I also include my evaluation of the treatment options, as I know that can be an especially challenging thing for IBS patients to do.

If you're pressed for time, just flip through and look at the tables. If you're not, feel free to read everything.

# How can you be sure you have IBS?

IBS is a diagnosis of exclusion. If you don't have other conditions that can also cause stomach problems, then you probably have IBS.

Most doctors skip straight to diagnosing IBS without thoroughly checking whether you might have these other conditions. That's unfortunate, because, unlike IBS, some of these other conditions actually have cures. If you're diagnosed correctly, your IBS could be solved a lot quicker.

Also, some of these conditions are much more serious than IBS. So, you definitely want to make sure you don't have these other conditions, because, if you do, you'll need to start treating them ASAP.

Here's a pretty exhaustive list of conditions that mimic IBS. Each row is a separate condition. Use it to potentially diagnose yourself. You'll need laboratory tests to confirm whether you're correct, but at least you'll be able to advocate for yourself at the doctor's office.

Note that the more of these conditions that you have, the more likely the diagnosis is. So, if you take the first example, an obese smoker on prednisone with constipation is more likely to have diverticulitis than a skinny non-smoker with diarrhea.

Also, please note that I've *italicized* the most important parts of a diagnosis. For example, unexplained weight loss is a pretty big warning sign for colon cancer and Chron's. If you just have diarrhea and don't have unexplained weight loss, neither colon cancer or Crohn's are likely (but they're still possible).

# IBS Diagnosis Table

| If you have | Or if you are | Then you might have |
|---|---|---|
| Bloating OR constipation OR diarrhea OR *bright blood in your stool* | Obese OR a smoker OR a user of anti-inflammatories/steroids | Diverticulitis |
| Constipation OR diarrhea OR *unexplained weight loss* OR fatigue | *Over the age of 45 (especially over the age of 65) OR have a history of cancer* | Colon cancer |
| *Bloody diarrhea* | | Ulcerative colitis |
| Diarrhea OR unexplained anemia OR *fever* OR *unexplained weight loss* OR growth retardation | | Crohn's disease |
| Joint pain OR *cold intolerance* OR constipation OR depression OR heavy menstrual flow OR unexplained weight gain or *fatigue* OR hair loss | *Female* | Hypothyroidism |
| Diarrhea AND nausea OR vomiting OR weight loss | *In an area with poor water quality or food hygiene standards* | Giardia |
| Abdominal bloating OR gas OR distension OR diarrhea | *A user of proton pump inhibitors (e.g. Prilosec) OR opioids OR gastric bypass OR colectomy* | Small intestinal bacterial overgrowth (SIBO) |
| Diarrhea OR bloating OR fatigue OR anemia OR *unexplained blisters (dermatitis herpetiformis)* | *Type 1 diabetic* | Celiac disease |

| Symptoms | Risk factors | Condition |
| --- | --- | --- |
| *Diarrhea* | | Bile acid malabsorption |
| *Constipation* | *Over 65* OR *African American* OR *pregnant/a mother* | Dyssnergic defecation |
| Abdominal pain and bloating OR gas OR watery stool *following the ingestion of foods containing lactose* | Black, Latino, or *Asian* | Lactose intolerance |
| Diarrhea OR constipation OR brain fog OR joint/muscle pain, OR skin rash/dermatitis | Female OR in the third to fourth decade of life | Non celiac gluten sensitivity |
| Nausea and vomiting OR *feeling of fullness or burning in your stomach* OR blood in your vomit or stool. | *In an area with poor water quality or food hygiene standards* | H. pylori |
| Constipation OR diarrhea OR nausea OR *a feeling of early fullness* | | A motility disorder |
| Constipation OR sense of a blockage during defecation OR *bladder pain* OR *abnormal urination* OR *pelvic ache after intercourse* OR pelvic pain unrelated to intercourse | Female OR have *injury to pelvic floor from surgery, trauma, or long-term damage (i.e. bad posture)* | Pelvic floor dysfunction |
| Constipation AND *poor response to laxatives* | Elderly OR female OR have history of sexual abuse | Slow-transit constipation |

| Constipation AND unexplained weight loss OR *constant thirst* OR *frequent urination* | *Pregnant* OR *obese* | Type I diabetes, type II diabetes, gestational diabetes |
| --- | --- | --- |
| Constipation OR *shuffling walk* OR *loss of smell* OR sleep disturbance | *Over 65* OR exposed to chemicals/herbicides in youth | Parkinson's |
| Constipation OR nausea OR *feel full early (early satiety)* | *Diabetic* OR obese | Gastroparesis |
| Constipation OR *pain/loss of vision in one eye over hours or days* OR *shooting pains down your arms or legs* OR *muscular weakness* | | Multiple sclerosis |
| Diarrhea OR *any sort of allergies* | | Mast cell related conditions |

****RARE CONDITIONS FOLLOW BELOW (you probably don't have these)****

| *Constipation since early childhood* | | Hirschsprung's disease |
| --- | --- | --- |
| Chronic or intermittent watery diarrhea OR unexplained weight loss, OR joint pain | *Over 65* OR *female* | Microscopic colitis |

| | | |
|---|---|---|
| *Flushing* OR diarrhea OR *shortness of breath* OR *palpitation* | | Carcinoid syndrome (part of carcinoid tumors) |
| Nausea OR vomiting, OR diarrhea OR anemia OR weight loss | | Eosinophilic gastroenteritis |
| *Kidney problems* AND anorexia OR constipation | *On dialysis* | Uremia |

# Steps to treat IBS

If you've made it through the whole list above and none of those apply to you, you probably just have IBS.

It's more likely you have IBS if you have a history of anxiety or depression, are female, or especially if you've *recently had a stomach bug*.

Now you're looking for treatment. Good on you! My recommendations are to start with a food restriction diet. Take away everything but chicken and rice, then slowly add the rest back in.

If you have diarrhea, you might try a low FODMAP diet, eating small, regular portions, and/or limiting gassy foods like beans, cabbages, and onions.

If you have constipation, you might try psyllium or linseed.

If you want to try medication, I'd recommend very high doses of cholecalciferol (Vitamin D3), like 50k IU every 2 weeks. You might also try peppermint oil for short term diarrhea relief.

That's my short list. For my long list, including evaluation and limitations of treatments, read on!

# IBS Treatment Table

| Potential IBS treatment | Evaluation | Limitations |
| --- | --- | --- |
| Low FODMAP for diarrhea and constipation | Low FODMAP diets seem to work. | The studies are only 1-3 months. It's not clear what happens if you resume a normal diet after that time span.<br><br>Low FODMAP diets doesn't necessarily work better than just eating normal portions at regular times and reducing fat, insoluble fibers, caffeine, beans, cabbages, and onions. It works better if you have diarrhea. |
| Exercise for constipation | Works well | |
| Gluten free diet (for non celiac) | It can work, but there's not a big effect. | It only works for people who are sensitive to gluten (it's not for anyone with IBS). |

| Fiber for constipation | Ispaghula (psyllium) and linseed, which are soluble fibers, are probably effective in all forms of IBS.<br><br>Linseed seems like it's probably better than psyllium. | All studies were done over a max of 1-3 months.<br><br>The studies aren't very well designed.<br><br>Bran and insoluble fiber are probably not effective in any form of IBS. |
| --- | --- | --- |
| Anti spasmodics (dicyclomine, peppermint oil, pinaverium, trimebutine) for diarrhea | They have ok effects for abdominal pain and bigger effects for overall symptom scores. | |
| Discontinuation of proton pump inhibitors for diarrhea | Not really a cure for IBS, but PPI overuse does lead to SIBO. | |
| Antidepressants for diarrhea and constipation | Antidepressants probably work if your IBS is caused by depression or anxiety. It's unclear whether they work if you don't. | Antidepressants aren't more effective in IBS than therapy.<br>It's unclear if the type of antidepressant matters, but it most likely varies from person to person. You'll need to experiment to find the best form for you. |
| Rifaximin for diarrhea and constipation | Rifaximin can definitely benefit IBS-D, and may help IBS-C. It doesn't seem to have any side effects. | |

| | | |
|---|---|---|
| Vitamin D3 for diarrhea | Very high doses of vitamin D every 2 weeks (50,000 IU) probably improve IBS symptoms. | Taking really high doses of vitamin D can cause side effects. If you get side effects, stop taking vitamin D. |
| Soy isoflavones for diarrhea | Soy isoflavones may improve IBS in women. | There aren't really good studies in men. There are no good long term studies either. |
| Acupuncture for diarrhea and constipation | Real acupuncture works just as well as fake acupuncture (having someone pretend to stick needles in you). Both work ok. | It's just a placebo effect, and there are probably cheaper ones. |
| Probiotics for diarrhea and constipation | Probiotics may have a small effect. | The type of bacteria in the probiotic and the formulation matters a lot, as a lot of probiotics are useless or destroyed in the stomach. It's not a cure all. |
| Mesalazine | Mesalazine is probably not effective in IBS. | |
| Loperamide | Loperamide is helpful for diarrhea and diarrhea-related symptoms. | There aren't great long-term studies. It may make pain at night worse. |
| Fecal microbiota transplant for diarrhea | Sometimes really helpful, sometimes not helpful at all. | Nasojejunal tube and colonoscopy seem like they work better than capsule for administration. |

| Antihistamines (e.g. cromolyn) for diarrhea | Works really well in patients with diarrhea, even if they normally would follow an elimination diet | Mild nausea is an occasional side effect |
| --- | --- | --- |
| ***Osmotic laxatives for constipation follow below*** | | |
| Polyethylene glycol (Miralax) for constipation | Works very well for chronic constipation. | Diarrhea as side effect, but goes away with a lower dose |
| Magnesium citrate powder | Works well as short-term constipation treatment | Can be dangerous if taken in high doses or over the long-term, or in patients with kidney problems. Generally not worth it. |
| Lactulose (cephulac) | Works ok. | Works worse than polyethylene glycol. |
| Linaclotide (Linzess) | Works ok in chronic constipation. | Diarrhea is a very common side effect. By prescription only. |

| | | |
|---|---|---|
| ***Stimulant laxatives follow below*** | | |
| Bisacodyl (Dulcolax) | Works well for chronic constipation. | Diarrhea is very common. Long-term use often leads to "addiction", in which you have to use bisacodyl to poop and it takes a while to become "unaddicted". |
| Senna/sennosides (Ex-lax) | Works well for immediate release of constipation. | Results in intense diarrhea. Long-term use leads to blisters on the butthole. |
| ***Atypical laxatives follow below*** | | |
| Lubiprostone (Amitiza), which increases intestinal fluid secretion | Works well for chronic constipation and quickly. | Nausea is a common side effect. |
| Prucalopride (Motegrity), a highly selective 5-HT 4 receptor agonist (neurotransmitter in the gut) | Works well in constipation and gastroparesis | Nausea is common and can be severe |

| Plecanatide (Trulance), a selective 5-HT 4 receptor agonist | Works ok in constipation. Very low amount of side effects compared to other atypical laxatives. | |
|---|---|---|
| ***Surgeries follow below*** | | |
| Total abdominal colectomy with ileorectal anastomosis (TAC IRA) | Reasonably effective treatment for colonic inertia | Semi-frequent diarrhea is very common as a long-term side effect |
| Laparoscopic total colectomy | Effective treatment for colonic inertia that's less invasive than TAC IRA, with greater satisfaction (around 80%) | Has only been done on women. Semi-frequent diarrhea is very common as a long-term side effect |

## A note on stimulant vs osmotic laxatives

A lot of people are scared of stimulant laxatives and will literally never try them.

This is a mistake for two reasons. First, stimulant laxatives can be effective in situations where osmotic laxatives are not. If constipation is making you miserable and osmotic laxatives have not worked, then you should not choose being constipated forever over trying osmotic laxatives.

Second, the reason why people get surgery for constipation is because they do not respond to any laxatives whatsoever, usually because they have complete colonic inertia. Whatever kind of total colectomy you get (TAC IRA or laparoscopic), it is a serious surgery. It is better to rely on stimulant laxatives than to get the surgery if you have that option.

# Dealing with your doctor

Once you've made your way through the diagnosis table and come up with a few ideas of what might be wrong with your digestive system, you'll likely need to go to the doctor to confirm and get most treatments.

Here's some advice on your journey.

## Your family doctor/GP/NP

Your first stop is going to be at a generalist. This might be someone called a family doctor, a general practitioner, or a nurse practitioner.

These people are not going to know a lot about your condition. They received a bit of training in school on this topic, and that's pretty much it. Their job is to make sure you don't have any really common conditions, then send you on your way to a specialist. In other words, they are gatekeepers.

Your best plan of attack here is to do the tests they ask, get paper and digital copies of all the tests and records that they generate, then politely but firmly request to be referred out to a specialist in your insurance network. Your insurance will probably have a list of specialists in your network, which will help with this last step.

Some of them, unfortunately, also seem to regard it as their job to prevent you from getting to a specialist. This might come in the form of telling you that your condition is normal, untreatable, or all in your head. Now, it's undeniable that mental health affects digestive health: everyone's had the experience of a queasy stomach before going on stage, or being unable to poop at a friend's house.

However, in my experience, general practitioners are way, way too eager to ascribe every digestive problem as a mental health problem. Don't treat this as a medical fact! Again, they do NOT know a lot about your condition, or any digestive conditions. Just nod when they say this, and politely ask to be referred to a specialist.

### Tests to be done at your general practitioner

1. **Standard metabolic panel**: this is a test of blood levels of common functions. The findings here don't apply to digestive health for the most part, unless your blood levels for something are crazy. In that case, you're in for a very different experience than normal IBS sufferers.

2. **Celiac blood panel:** if you have diarrhea, they'll probably want you to get a celiac blood panel to check for antibodies against gluten. This is a pretty accurate test for celiac, so it's definitely useful if celiac's disease is at all a concern.

3. **Fecal occult blood test:** the "occult" part of this sounds spooky, but it just means that it's a test for hidden blood in your feces. As you can see from the diagnostic table, blood in feces is a big sign of inflammatory bowel diseases, so this is a useful test to make sure you don't have one of those.

## Your gastroenterologist

Your next stop after your GP is your gastro.

Now, the good news is that gastros have way more experience and knowledge of gastrointestinal disorders than your GP. The bad news is that still doesn't mean you can take your hands off the steering wheel and just assume the gastro knows best. You still need to do your research, ask pointed questions, and keep paper and digital copies of all the tests and records they generate.

Why? Well, because gastros have a lot of experience with the most common intestinal disorders, and less experience with the less common intestinal disorders. Likewise, they have a lot of experience with the most common treatments, and less experience with the least common treatments.

So, if you have a common disorder and need a common treatment, they will likely be able to help you a lot better than if you have an uncommon disorder or need an uncommon treatment.

If you do have an uncommon disorder, like total colonic inertia or microscopic colitis, you will either need a gastro with experience in that specific disorder or you will need to be very in charge of your health. Don't be afraid to ask if your gastro has experience in that specific disorder, either! They tend to accept patients even when they don't have experience treating that specific disorder, and it's not fun being someone's first colonic inertia patient.

You will also need to be very in charge of your health if you have a condition that requires other specialist doctors besides gastros, like Parkinson's or multiple sclerosis. Doctors are bad at interfacing across specialties. Your GP is supposed to be the one to make sure that your neurologist talks to your gastro, but your GP might drop the ball. Keep your records and make sure they ok your treatments with one another.

Finally, it's worth noting that some old school gastros are also way, way too eager to ascribe digestive problems to mental health. I once talked to a gastro who proudly told me about the experiments he used to run to find out people who were "faking" non-celiac gluten sensitivity. This was *after* I told him I was sensitive to gluten. You have to pity his gluten sensitive patients who were told that they were, essentially, drama queens.

### Tests to be done at the gastro

[Note: there are a lot of tests that could be done, depending on your specific suspected condition. These are just some of them.]

1. **Stool cultures**: you give them a sample of your poop, they see if you have parasites like Giardia or H. pylori. Especially useful for people with diarrhea.
2. **SIBO:** you drink a kind of gross sweet drink, they test to see if there are bacteria in your small intestines snacking on the drink. Again, useful for people with diarrhea.
3. **Comprehensive thyroid panel**: note the <u>comprehensive</u> portion of this. You want to see if there are any possible hypothyroid issues (or hyperthyroid issues) that could be causing your digestive issues. This is more useful for constipation, but still useful for diarrhea.
4. **Endoscopy with small bowel aspirate and biopsy**: this is a more serious test, because it requires sedation. It tests for inflammatory bowel diseases, and an eosinophilia biopsy to check for allergies. Useful for anyone with suspected inflammatory bowel diseases.
5. **SITZ Marker Study (a.ka. a motility test)**: this is a useful but somewhat rare test for anyone with chronic constipation that doesn't respond to laxatives. It checks to see which, if any, parts of your large intestine aren't working properly.
6. **Anorectal manometry**: this is a test for anyone who may have rectal problems, like chronic constipation or fecal incontinence. They put a tube in your butt and measure how well your rectum squeezes and relaxes, to see if your problems might lie in your rectum.
7. **Magnetic resonance defecography**: they use magnetic resonance imaging (MRI) to watch what your body does internally when you poop to see if there are obvious mechanical issues. This does require an MRI machine, which are long, loud metal tubes that you'll have to lie in for 30 minutes to an hour. This is most useful for constipation.
8. **Serum tryptase:** this is a blood test used to check for mast cell activation. It's a little complicated to interpret, and definite results require more invasive and expensive tests, like bone marrow tests and urine tests. It's most useful for people with diarrhea.

# The science of diarrhea and constipation

At the end of the day, both diarrhea and constipation are conditions where something's gone wrong in the digestive system. If we want to understand how things go wrong, first we'll have to understand how digestion is supposed to work.

Digestion is supposed to work in three phases: in the mouth, in the stomach, and in the intestines. At the end, the food passes out of the intestines, past your rectum, and into your toilet bowl.

In the mouth, the first thing that needs to happen is the food needs to be broken down so it can be swallowed. Chewing is the most obvious part of this. Another part of this is the digestive enzymes in saliva, which also help digesting food. Once the food is chewed enough, the saliva and the tongue helps the food slide down into the esophagus. From this moment on, all the food's movement will be done by involuntary waves of muscles called peristalsis, slowly shuffling the food from one stage to the next.

So far, so good. Very few people with digestive problems have problems with these steps, and conditions that inhibit swallowing (like ALS) tend to cause much bigger problems than just simple digestion.

The food then needs to pass through the esophagus and down into the stomach. In order for this to happen, food needs to not pass into the lungs, and, ideally, no gastric acid comes up from the stomach back up into the esophagus, because that stuff is very harsh on soft tissue.

The way in which gastric acid is prevented from coming back up into the esophagus is the lower esophageal sphincter, a ring of muscle that closes off the bottom of the esophagus. When that ring of muscle doesn't close properly (or at the right time), you get "heartburn" or GERD.

Once the food makes its way into the stomach, gastric acid and enzymes start to digest it and turn it into a form that's usable by the body. Simultaneously, the stomach churns the food, mixing it with the acid and enzymes. This is also where amino acids are absorbed.

Again, this usually part of the process usually isn't an issue for people with digestive issues, except for people with gastroparesis. It's the next part that's the problem.

After this, the food passes into the small intestine. The small intestine is where the majority of nutrients in food gets absorbed. The first part of the small intestine is the duodenum, which holds food and prepares the rest of the small intestine to start digesting it. The second part is the jejunum, which digests all the easy stuff (basically everything except fats). The last part is the ileum, which digests the difficult stuff and also recycles the bile salts.

There are a lot of problems that can go wrong at literally any stage in the small intestine:

1. Celiac disease, which is an immune response to gluten, causes cracks and grooves in the duodenum, making it difficult for the duodenum to hold food and prepare the small intestine.

2. Lactose intolerance is when lactase, the lactose digesting enzyme, is lacking from the jejunum, which makes the small intestine skip digesting lactose, so the lactose gets digested in the colon and causes gas buildup.

3. Crohn's can cause ulceration anywhere, but often causes ulceration in the ileum, which is why it's difficult for Crohn's patients to digest fats.

4. Last, small intestinal bacterial overgrowth (SIBO) is when bacteria makes its way up to the small intestines from the large intestines or colon, messing up the digestive process.

But, even if things do go wrong, eventually the food does make its way past the small intestine and into the large intestine. At this point, the food is mostly digested and there's not a ton left. What is left is water, salts, and really difficult to digest material, like fiber. So, what's left to do is to get the remaining water, salts, and anything worth digesting out of the food, and evacuate the rest of it. The digestion is done in the colon, the evacuation is done through the rectum and out the anal canal.

The colon consists of six parts: the cecum, the ascending colon, the transverse colon, the descending colon, the sigmoid colon, and the rectum. Why so many? Well, frankly, it's just a very long tube packed into a small space that requires a long time to do its digestion. This is pretty much the only workable way to get all the digestion done that needs to be done.

The colon doesn't do all its work itself, by the way. The colon does its water and salt absorption by itself, but there are tons of bacteria in the colon to help with digestion of the really difficult stuff. Most of the digestion done by these bacteria is helpful. For example, the bacteria create thiamine, which we need for our brain. No thiamine results in lots of bad problems, like derangement.

Unfortunately, sometimes the digestion is unhelpful. The bacteria digest whatever they come in contact with. In doing so, they can create gas or unpleasant byproducts. That's what happens with FODMAPS, for example.

You can probably already tell that a lot of things can go wrong in the colon. If food gets rushed along the colon for any reason, there's not enough time to absorb the water and you get diarrhea. Meanwhile, if food moves through too slowly, too much water gets absorbed and the food gets dry and impacted, so you get constipation. That's how loperamide (Imodium) works, by the way: it slows down the muscles of the colon and lets the food spend more time in the colon.

Disruptions of the blood supply to the colon or colonic nerves can also cause major problems. Remember: all this food is moving by your own muscular movement. It's not moving itself. If the muscles don't work properly, the food gets stuck.

The last part of the colon is the rectum. This is the holding place for poop. It gets held in place there by anal sphincters, strong rings of muscle like the ones in your esophagus. Once there's enough pressure on the anal sphincters, the person feels the urge to poop. If there's a lot of pressure, they have to poop.

Any muscular or nervous problems here can result in a poorly functioning sphincter that either doesn't open up or doesn't close properly. These result in constipation or fecal incontinence, respectively. Ulcerative colitis, on the other hand, results in ulcers here, which can be unpleasant or even dangerous (it's really not good to have poop piling up near a hole that goes directly to your bloodstream).

Finally, there's the anal canal and the anus. These parts we're all reasonably familiar with. These anus is helped by cushions that make passage of stool easier. Problems with these cushions can cause inflammation or bleeding, which is commonly known as hemorrhoids.

And thus concludes our brief tour of the digestive system. I hope you enjoyed it.

Now let's relate our conditions to what can go wrong.

# What goes wrong with your digestion

Lots of things can go wrong in your digestion. It's a complicated, multi-hour, multi-step process, one in which you ingest literally anything from the outside world and your body has to make energy from it.

I mean, seriously, have you ever seen a little kid stuffing things in his mouth? His digestive system has to make sense of incoming food, dirt, bacteria, and probably pennies. From that, it has to sort through what's useful, transform the useful parts into usable energy, get rid of any unhelpful parts, and destroy or kick out any invaders that have hitched a ride.

It's a wonder our digestive system works as well as it does. It's a hard job! The list below details a few of the ways in which your digestive system can mess up, with the understanding that we still appreciate our digestive system for all it does and can do.

1. **Diverticulitis:** diverticulitis comes from hernias of the colon, which means that the blood vessels underneath the skin of the colon burst through the walls. This makes it easy for them to bleed, and also makes your colon work worse (because there's a blood vessel where there's supposed to be the outer layer of the colon). This usually results in diarrhea and blood in the stool.
2. **Ulcerative colitis**: as mentioned, these are holes in your colon, caused by your immune system attacking your colon. This can have a variety of bad consequences, because digested food/poop ends up stuck in places it shouldn't. Also, your colon works worse, causing food to pass through quickly and resulting in diarrhea.
3. **Crohn's disease**: this is closely related to UC, except it's general inflammation throughout the digestive tract. When your gastrointestinal tract is inflamed, your body treats that as a warning sign to evacuate everything from the area so it can fix the problem. For people with Crohn's, this evacuation command is happening all the time, and the body is occasionally sending immune system "troops" to destroy whatever's there. Unfortunately, that's your digestive tract, leading to ulcers.
4. **Hypothyroidism**: this happens when your body doesn't produce enough thyroid hormone. Hormones are very general bodily signals. The thyroid hormone gives a general bodily signal for your tissues and organs to do more and speed up: more heat, higher heart rate, more energy production. Low levels of thyroid hormones means that your body is slower than it should, including your digestion, leading to constipation.
5. **Giardia**: Giardia is a parasite that likes to take up residence in the surface of your small intestine, raise a family, and settle in. This makes your small intestine work much worse, and the digestion process gets messed up. Food just passes through your digestive tract instead of getting absorbed, and you get violent diarrhea.
6. **Small intestinal bacterial overgrowth**: as mentioned, SIBO is when the bacteria from your colon take up residence in your small intestine. They start digesting food in your small intestine and release gas. Your small intestine isn't equipped to handle the gas production, and you feel bloated.
7. **Celiac disease**: celiac disease is an immune reaction to gluten. Normally, your small intestine passes wheat through so it can be digested in the large intestine. In celiac, your small

intestine has tiny gaps in its surface, and little parts of gluten get stuck in there. Once your immune system notices, it freaks out because it thinks there's an invader in your small intestine. It launches a full scale war to destroy the invader, and your small intestine gets caught in the crossfire.

8. **Bile acid malabsorption**: as mentioned, fats are hard to digest. So, your liver produces bile acids or bile salts to help digest them. The way it's supposed to work is that these caustic chemicals are produced in the liver, used in the small intestine, taken up again in the ileum, and recycled to be used again. In bile acid malabsorption, either the ileum doesn't take up the bile acids well enough or the liver overproduces bile acids. Either way, you end up with too much bile acid in your large intestine, irritating everything and causing diarrhea as your body just dumps the bile acid out.

9. **Dyssynergic defecation:** this is a purely muscular problem. Basically, the way you poop is supposed to be relaxing the rectum, pushing out through the anal canal, relaxing the anus, and then the poop gets pushed out. People with dyssynergic defecation, for whatever reason, mess this process up, often by contracting the anus instead of relaxing it. So, they end up being bad at pooping, and they get constipated.

10. **Lactose intolerance**: as mentioned, lactose intolerance is when the needed enzyme for digesting lactose, namely lactase, isn't there. So the bacteria in your large intestine digest it instead, produce gas, and give you diarrhea. It's worth noting that almost all mammals (and a large proportion of humanity) loses the ability to produce lactase after childhood. It's the weird ones who still keep it.

11. **H. pylori**: H. pylori is a bacteria that takes up residence in the stomach by burrowing into the surface and then creating urease to protect itself from stomach acidity. If there's just a few H. pylori, they aren't really noticeable. If, for whatever reason, they start reproducing rapidly, suddenly you've got a lot of little holes in your stomach, and that's not good. You get blood in your poop and a bad feeling in your stomach.

12. **Pelvic floor dysfunction**: ever seen a skeleton? You'll notice they have an empty space between their hip bones. The only reason why our organs, like our intestines, don't fall out between that empty space is because our muscles occupy the space instead and hold everything up. If those muscles stop working as well (e.g. because of the trauma of childbirth), the organs stop being held up as well, and the careful organization of our digestive organs becomes a mess. For example, it is really hard to control your poop if your rectum is below your anus.

13. **Slow transit constipation/colonic inertia**: as mentioned, the only way food moves through your digestive tract after you swallow it is by muscular contractions. Interruptions to the nerves or blood supply of these digestive tract muscles means that food moves more slowly or even not at all through the digestive tract.

14. **Diabetes**: diabetes, whether type I, type II, or another type, is characterized by something being messed up with insulin. Insulin is another hormone, and it's generally responsible for telling the body to start using glucose as fuel. Low levels of insulin are interpreted by the body to use fat as fuel instead, usually when there's not enough glucose to go around. If this signal gets messed up, the body burns fat when it already has a ton of glucose in the bloodstream, and the excess glucose gets in the way of a lot of bodily processes, including digestion.

15. **Parkinson's**: Parkinson's is a disease where the body stops producing dopamine. Dopamine is both a neurotransmitter and a hormone. As a hormone, it has complex effects on the digestive system, but seems to work by having the digestive system speed up. Lack of dopamine causes the digestive system to slow down, causing constipation.

16. **Gastroparesis**: gastroparesis is when your stomach's muscle contractions don't work well (often due to nerve damage), so the stomach's digestive juices never get mixed well with the food. This makes digestion work more slowly and worse, because the intestines get food that's not really digested yet. This backs up the digestive system, and makes it hard for people to eat more because the old food is being digested super slowly.

17. **Multiple sclerosis**: multiple sclerosis is a disease in which the sheaths of neurons (the myelin) break down. These sheaths have two functions: protection of the neuron, and allowing electrical impulses to jump from myelin sheath to myelin sheath, instead of traveling down the "wire". When these break down, all sorts of nervous system problems develop, including digestive issues.

18. **Hirschsprung's disease**: nerves are missing from a part of the colon, so the muscles don't work there and food gets stuck. The traditional way to fix it is just to cut out that part of the colon and surgically reattach the other parts.

19. **Microscopic colitis**: microscopic colitis is another case in which immune system cells infiltrate the colon (notice a pattern?) In this case, there's a bunch of them causing lots of little local collateral damage, but no big collateral damage. This results in microscopic colonic inflammation.

20. **Carcinoid syndrome**: carcinoid syndrome happens after carcinoid tumors. Carcinoid tumors are tumors that occur in your hormonal system. If the tumors make their way to your colon, they can accidentally release a bunch of hormones called vasodilators. These vasodilators tell your digestive system to speed up continually, giving you diarrhea.

21. **Eosinophilic gastroenteritis**: yet another case in which the immune system infiltrates the gastrointestinal tract.  In this one, however, it's usually the stomach, and the specific immune system cells are eosinophils, which are responsible for a lot of autoimmune diseases, including some severe types of asthma.

22. **Uremia**: uremia means you have high levels of urea in the bloodstream, which is bad. Urea is supposed to be urinated out (hence the name), and high levels of urea means your urinary system isn't working, which probably means your kidneys are really messed up. Your kidneys do a lot of things, but one of the big ones is maintaining water levels in your body, which is also a big function of digestion. Broken kidneys means broken water levels, so your intestines absorb too much water and give you constipation.

23. **Mast cell activation syndrome:** your mast cells trigger rapid generalized immune responses. You might know them from such hits as "Is that pollen or a deadly invader? Don't know, but let's sneeze violently to avoid having to figure it out!". They can do similar things in your digestive system: if they're not sure if something's an invader in the digestive system, mast cells will trigger diarrhea to get the invader out. In our sanitized world, our mast cells tend to be unfamiliar with what actual pathogens look like, and, as a result, are on a hair trigger, causing diarrhea for harmless food items.

# The science of fixing what goes wrong with your digestive system

There are a lot of different treatments for IBS and IBS-related issues. It may be a mystery to you how some of them work, or why some work and others don't. This list explores the treatments that do work and explains why they work, using our knowledge from before.


1. **Low FODMAP diets**: FODMAP stands for fermentable oligosaccharides, disaccharides, monosaccharides, and polyols. These are difficult to digest carbohydrates that don't get digested in the small intestine. So, the bacteria in the large intestine digest them. When the bacteria in the large intestine digest them, they produce gas as a byproduct, which can interfere with digestion or force food along more quickly than it would be otherwise. As we know, food moving too quickly causes diarrhea.

2. **Exercise**: exercise is broadly useful for a lot of conditions. Constipation is one of them, because the jostling from exercise can physically help food digest, and the increased blood flow from your pumping heart can let the muscles in your digestive tract work more efficiently. In order for any muscles to work, they need blood flow to carry energy to them and carry waste products away from them. More blood flow means, broadly, more efficient muscles.

3. **Gluten free diet (for non celiac)**: it's not entirely clear why this works. It may be related to the autoimmune issues of celiac sufferers, which is when the immune system attacks small pieces of gluten that get stuck in the digestive tract. Or, it might be related to FODMAP diets, where grains get digested in the large intestine by bacteria and we get gas as a byproduct.

4. **Fiber**: soluble fiber is fiber that dissolves in water. The easiest way to understand why it works is literally just to put it in a bowl and pour water on it, then watch as it becomes a sludge. It absorbs water in the digestive system, gluing whatever's around it and allowing it to slide smoothly through the digestive tract. It also slides relatively slowly (because it's viscous), which is why it can be helpful in diarrhea as well. Insoluble fiber is supposed to work by scraping the walls of the large intestine and triggering the secretion of mucus, which would let the food slide more smoothly, but it doesn't seem to actually help much.

5. **Antispasmodics**: antispasmodics work in a variety of ways, but all of them slow down the movement of the intestines. I'll take peppermint oil as a specific example. Peppermint oil blocks calcium channels in the intestinal muscles. Calcium channels are how muscles signal to contract. Peppermint oil stops the signalling, which means the intestinal muscles don't contract. So food just sits there, like you've temporarily given yourself colonic inertia.

6. **Discontinuation of proton pump inhibitors for SIBO**: proton pump inhibitors stop the secretion of gastric acid. This is good for people with too much gastric acid, like those with heartburn. Unfortunately, fear of gastric acid is a big reason why large intestine bacteria don't make their way up to the small intestine. When you take that gastric acid away, the bacteria move in.

7. **Antidepressants for diarrhea and constipation**: one of the really common ways that antidepressants work is by messing with the supply of serotonin in your body. Serotonin is primarily used as a neurotransmitter in the brain, but it's also reused as a signaller in the gut as a contraction signal. More serotonin promotes more contraction, which promotes faster movement through the digestive tract. Your body has a lot of control mechanisms for levels of hormones and neurotransmitters, though, to stop them from getting too high, which is likely why this mechanism doesn't work as well as would be ideal.

8. **Rifaximin:** rifaximin is primarily an antibiotic that physically interferes with bacteria reproducing by binding to their RNA. RNA, if you remember from bio, is a set of instructions on how to make more cells, or, in this case, bacterial cells. Rifaximin attaches itself to the instructions and makes them unreadable. The bacteria don't know how to make more of themselves, they die out, and any bacterial problems in your gut are lessened.

9. **Vitamin D3:** Vitamin D is somewhat hard to explain. It does many, many things in the body, which is why people try it as a cure for everything. Broadly speaking, it reduces inflammation, which is why it can be helpful for inflamed guts. Specifically speaking, it's much harder to tell.

10. **Soy isoflavones**: isoflavones can, in some circumstances, look enough like estrogen for the body to mistake one for the other. Estrogen can have an impact on the gut, as anyone with a monthly cycle can tell you. If isoflavones have any effect, it probably has something to do with that.

11. **Acupuncture and other placebos**: acupuncture is purely a placebo effect, which is why fake acupuncture works as well as real acupuncture. Placebo effects can do wonders for pain and anxiety, because pain and anxiety do occur in the brain. This is why children stop crying when their parents kiss their scraped knee. Any parts of IBS related to pain and anxiety can be helped by this sort of placebo.

12. **Probiotics**: probiotics are pretty sketchy, to be honest. The idea is that IBS is caused by messed up populations of bacteria in the gut, which seems reasonable enough. However, it is actually pretty hard to get bacteria to form colonies in the gut if they don't want to: just ask scientists in a lab about how temperamental bacteria are about growing in petri dishes. Also, I don't think anyone knows what the "ideal bacterial gut colony" is like.

13. **Loperamide**: loperamide is technically an opioid. Much like serotonin, opioid receptors are present not only in the brain, but all over the body. Opioids do the opposite of serotonin, though: they tell the body to relax, including the gut. The relaxation response also explains the other, better known effects of opioids.

14. **Cromolyn**: it's actually unclear why cromolyn works. It may work by inhibiting chloride channels, which are widely used as regulatory mechanisms throughout the body. This somehow prevents mast cells from releasing their chemicals that provoke the evacuation response.

15. **Polyethylene glycol (Miralax)**: polyethylene glycol is a chemical that loves water. It will bind as much as it can and carry it with itself. Along with its many other uses, this makes it an excellent osmotic laxative, as, when it hits the large intestines, it has a lot of water with it.

16. **Magnesium citrate powder:** magnesium undergoes a number of chemical changes in the intestines. By the time it reaches its final form, magnesium carbonate, it's created a steep osmotic gradient. Like water traveling up a dry paper towel, water in the intestines goes towards the magnesium carbonate, relieving constipation.

17. **Lactulose:** lactulose, as a complex sugar, gets metabolized by bacteria in the large intestine. The first byproduct of this is gas. The second is a decreased pH of the large intestine, which results in expansion of the intestine. The two of these combined make you have to poop.

18. **Linaclotide (Linzess)**: linaclotide targets a very specific receptor, guanylate cyclase 2C. This is one of the receptors the body relies on to know whether there's a foreign invader in the digestive tract. Linaclotide agonizes that receptor, the body gets convinced there's an invader, and the digestive tract is evacuated.

19. **Bisacodyl (Dulcolax)**: bisacodyl works by directly stimulating the muscles of the colon, and by promoting the increase of salt in the colon, which water then follows. It's unclear how exactly it stimulates the muscles.

20. **Senna (Ex-Lax):** senna also directly stimulates the muscles, but it's unclear how.

21. **Lubiprostone (Amitiza):** lubiprostone also activates chloride channels, but, in this case on the intestinal surface itself. This makes the surface secrete a chloride fluid, which allows stool to move along.

22. **Prucalopride (Motegrity):** prucalopride is another one that affects serotonin, but, in this case, it activates the serotonin receptors directly.

23. **Plecanatide (Trulance):** plecanatide does the same thing, but a little less directly.

24. **Total abdominal colectomy with ileorectal anastomosis:** they cut open your stomach, snip out the offending parts, and staple the non offending parts to each other.

25. **Laparoscopic total colectomy:** same as previous, but instead of making a big cut, they make a tiny cut and sneak a camera through. This is a bit safer and allows for faster recovery.

# Evidence

## How I evaluated the evidence

Evaluating evidence is hard in general, and evaluating evidence in IBS is no exception.

I'll list out those problems, then list how I tried to solve them.

First, there are specific IBS issues.

IBS has a variety of symptoms associated with it, and a treatment that fixes diarrhea will not necessarily fix constipation. This makes treatments difficult to measure in effectiveness. Some scientists try to make up for this by asking patients questions like, "Is your pain reduced?" or "Are you happy with your bowel movements?", but those can be biased by treatments that treat only pain or depression without affecting IBS-specific symptoms.

To solve this, I tried to tease out the various effects that treatments had on different symptoms of IBS when I could. I paid especially close attention to questions that could be biased, which was a particular issue in antidepressants, as those will obviously make people happier with any treatment.

IBS is also, obviously, really hard to diagnose. One study found that 30% of people with IBS-D actually have bile acid malabsorption. If that's true, then 30% of the people in any IBS-D study don't have IBS. What exactly does the study measure, then?

I didn't have a good way of solving this, so I just hoped for the best.

IBS studies are also often reliant on patient compliance, especially when testing dietary interventions like low FODMAP. This is...not great. This IBD study found only 55% diet compliance (i.e. patients ate different food than prescribed almost half of the time). From my own experience, I had a girlfriend who did weight loss studies. Even when the study gave her food to take home, she would throw it out and just eat her own food because it tasted better. Needless to say, she did not tell the clinicians this.

I tried to solve this by avoiding studies that were reliant on patient compliance and self-reporting. If I couldn't avoid the studies, I relied on them less for my recommendations.

So, those are some IBS specific issues. Let's talk about issues in general.

The gold standard for a trial is placebo-controlled, double-blind and randomized. Placebo-controlled means that half the people get a fake treatment, so the experimenters can weed out any people who would have gotten better regardless of if they got the control.

Double blind means that neither the patient nor the experimenters know whether they are getting a real treatment, so nobody can cheat on their measurements or reports if they have a belief one way or another. Last, randomized means people get randomly assigned to placebo or treatment, so we end up with the same sorts of people in both groups.

Reaching that gold standard is easier in some trials than in others. If we're testing a treatment like gluten, it's actually surprisingly easy if the experimenters are up for it. They just give every group a pill, and sometimes the pill contains wheat flour, sometimes rice flour. The experimenters don't know which pills are which until all the measurements are done.

However, if we're testing a treatment like low FODMAP, it's impossible. Everyone knows which diet is the low FODMAP diet. There's no faking it for either side. So, if a patient really believes low FODMAP will work for them, they might be a little more lax with their reports, (if they're between a 1 and 2 on a scale, they might choose 2 more often than 1). An experimenter might do the same.

I tried to notice when studies were falling away from the gold standard, but I don't want to just throw away all studies that don't reach that standard. Then I'd have to throw away a lot of potentially useful treatments. Instead, I weighed my judgments accordingly.

Once I was sure studies were performed well, I looked for consistently positive results. Any study can have a positive result once, especially if it's a small study, in the same way that it's easy to flip a coin 3 times and get all heads. But consistently getting heads when you flip a coin 100 times is a different story, and suggests there's actually something there.

I also looked for consistent results across measures. A treatment should improve IBS severity, overall satisfaction, and symptoms. If it only improves one measure, it suggests that measure might have been a fluke.

I also looked for big results in the form of big effect sizes vs. placebo. When there are treatments that can almost quadruple the effects of placebo like vitamin D, small effects like mesalazine which might work ok for some people didn't cut it.

Last, I combined all these together and got my evaluations.

## How I came up with my recommendations

Some technical notes on how to read these.

RR, which is relative risk, is basically the number with the bad outcome over the number with the good outcome. So, the smaller RR is, the better.

CI, which is the confidence interval, just accounts for error in the measurement. In the first study below, the RR is estimated to be 0.69, but it might be between 0.54 and 0.88.

I2 (which should really be $I^2$) is a measure of "heterogeneity", or how different the various effects are. The closer I2 gets to 100%, the greater the differences between studies (which makes you start to wonder why they're so different and if one study is messed up).

N, like n=39, is just how many patients there were in a specific group.

The P value, like P=0.62, is the likelihood that a difference found between treatments or conditions is a fluke. By convention, we use P<0.05 to mean significant, as in there's a less than 5% chance that the difference is a fluke.

[Note for statistics nerds: all the definitions above are rough definitions for a lay audience. If you know the definition better than that, then good on you! Please don't send me angry messages over it.]

My notes on each study are in *italics*.

**FODMAP**

*Low FODMAP diets seem to work, but the studies aren't very good. It doesn't necessarily work better than just eating regularly and reducing fat, insoluble fibers, caffeine, beans, cabbages, and onions. It works better if you have diarrhea.*

All studies were done over 1-3 months.

A Systematic Review and Meta-Analysis Evaluating the Efficacy of a Gluten-Free Diet and a Low FODMAPs Diet in Treating Symptoms of Irritable Bowel Syndrome - White Rose Research Online

*This is a meta-study for both gluten-free diet and low FODMAP. I used it to guide my thinking, but also looked at the studies myself.*

There were seven RCTs comparing a low FODMAP diet with various control interventions in 397 participants. A low FODMAP diet was associated with reduced global symptoms compared with control interventions (RR = 0.69; 95% CI 0.54 to 0.88; I2= 25%). The three RCTS that compared low FODMAP diet with rigorous control diets had the least heterogeneity between studies, but also the least magnitude of effect.

Diet Low in FODMAPs Reduces Symptoms of Irritable Bowel Syndrome as Well as Traditional Dietary Advice: A Randomized Controlled Trial - ScienceDirect

*Note that this study is relying on food diaries. This is an ok solution to problems of non compliance, but it's not great, as people can still lie or misremember. Keeping a food diet for 4 weeks is hard! Also, there's definitely an overlap between the low FODMAP diet and the normal diet. There's also no placebo group.*

Subjects were randomly assigned to groups that ate specific diets for 4 weeks—a diet low in FODMAPs (n = 38) or a diet frequently recommended for patients with IBS (ie, a regular meal pattern; avoidance of large meals; and reduced intake of fat, insoluble fibers, caffeine, and gas-producing foods, such as beans, cabbage, and onions), with greater emphasis on how and when to eat rather than on what foods to ingest (n = 37).

A total of 67 patients completed the dietary intervention (33 completed the diet low in FODMAPs, 34 completed the traditional IBS diet). The severity of IBS symptoms was reduced in both groups during the intervention ($P <$ .0001 in both groups before vs at the end of the 4-week diet), without a significant difference between the groups ($P =$ .62). At the end of the 4-week diet period, 19 patients (50%) in the low-FODMAP group had reductions in IBS severity scores ≥50 compared with baseline vs 17 patients (46%) in the traditional IBS diet group ($P =$ .72).

FODMAPs alter symptoms and the metabolome of patients with IBS: a randomised controlled trial | Gut (bmj.com)

*This study is looking directly at the metabolome, which is interesting, and should be more reliable than food diaries. The metabolome does seem to change a lot, which is interesting, but*

We performed a controlled, single blind study of patients with IBS (Rome III criteria) randomised to a low (n=20) or high (n=20) FODMAP diet for 3 weeks.

Thirty-seven patients (19 low FODMAP; 18 high FODMAP) completed the 3-week diet. The IBS-SSS was reduced in the low FODMAP diet group (p<0.001) but not the high FODMAP group. LBTs showed a minor decrease in H2 production in the low FODMAP compared with the high FODMAP group. Metabolic profiling of urine showed groups of patients with IBS differed significantly after the diet (p<0.01), with three metabolites (histamine, p-hydroxybenzoic acid, azelaic acid) being primarily responsible for discrimination between the two groups. Histamine, a measure of immune activation, was reduced eightfold in the low FODMAP group (p<0.05).

A Diet Low in FODMAPs Reduces Symptoms of Irritable Bowel Syndrome - ScienceDirect

*This is a pretty good study. They provided food and they collected stool instead of urine or self-report. Again, there's no placebo control, so that's a problem, but this is probably as good as you're going to get with a low FODMAP diet. I wish they had more people and over a longer term.*

In a study of 30 patients with IBS and 8 healthy individuals (controls, matched for demographics and diet), we collected dietary data from subjects for 1 habitual week. Participants then randomly were assigned to groups that received 21 days of either a diet low in FODMAPs or a typical Australian diet, followed by a washout period of at least 21 days, before crossing over to the alternate diet. Daily symptoms were rated using a 0- to 100-mm visual analogue scale. Almost all food was provided during the interventional diet periods, with a goal of less than 0.5 g intake of FODMAPs per meal for the low-FODMAP diet. All stools were collected from days 17–21 and assessed for frequency, weight, water content, and King's Stool Chart rating.

Subjects with IBS had lower overall gastrointestinal symptom scores (22.8; 95% confidence interval, 16.7–28.8 mm) while on a diet low in FODMAPs, compared with the Australian diet (44.9; 95% confidence interval, 36.6–53.1 mm; $P < .001$) and the subjects' habitual diet. Bloating, pain, and passage of wind also were reduced while IBS patients were on the low-FODMAP diet. Symptoms were minimal and unaltered by either diet among controls. Patients of all IBS subtypes had greater satisfaction with stool consistency while on the low-FODMAP diet, but diarrhea-predominant IBS was the only subtype with altered fecal frequency and King's Stool Chart scores.

**Gluten free diet (in non celiac)**

*Pretty good studies, but there's not a big effect. All studies were done over 1-3 months.*

A Systematic Review and Meta-Analysis Evaluating the Efficacy of a Gluten-Free Diet and a Low FODMAPs Diet in Treating Symptoms of Irritable Bowel Syndrome - White Rose Research Online

*Again, same meta review.*

Both selected patients that had already responded to a GFD, and then randomized them to continue the diet, or to have the diet "spiked" with gluten.

A GFD was associated with reduced global symptoms compared with a control diet (RR = 0.42; 95% CI 0.11 to 1.55; I2= 88%), although this was not statistically significant.

Gluten causes gastrointestinal symptoms in subjects without celiac disease: a double-blind randomized placebo-controlled trial - PubMed (nih.gov)

*Very skewed women:men ratio. This is "placebo controlled" with normal vs. gluten free muffins. It raises the question of whether the patients could tell the difference between the normal and gluten free muffins, which they probably could.*

A total of 34 patients (aged 29-59 years, 4 men) completed the study as per protocol. Overall, 56% had human leukocyte antigen (HLA)-DQ2 and/or HLA-DQ8. Adherence to diet and supplements was very high. Of 19 patients (68%) in the gluten group, 13 reported that symptoms were not adequately controlled compared with 6 of 15 (40%) on placebo (P=0.0001; generalized estimating equation). On a visual analog scale, patients were significantly worse with gluten within 1 week for overall symptoms (P=0.047), pain (P=0.016), bloating (P=0.031), satisfaction with stool consistency (P=0.024), and tiredness (P=0.001).

Non-Celiac Gluten Sensitivity Has Narrowed the Spectrum of Irritable Bowel Syndrome: A Double-Blind Randomized Placebo-Controlled Trial - PubMed (nih.gov)

*This one is a better placebo because they gave them gluten packets, which would be harder to tell taste wise from gluten free powder. However, the graphs, which I copied below, are terrible and clearly show overlap between placebo and gluten. I'm not a huge fan of this study or how they presented their information, but there does seem to be some effect.*

. In the second stage after six weeks, patients whose symptoms improved to an acceptable level were randomly divided into two groups; patients either received packages containing powdered gluten (35 cases) or patients received placebo (gluten free powder) (37 cases). Overall, the symptomatic improvement was statistically different in the gluten-containing group compared with placebo group in 9 (25.7%), and 31 (83.8%) patients respectively (p < 0.001).

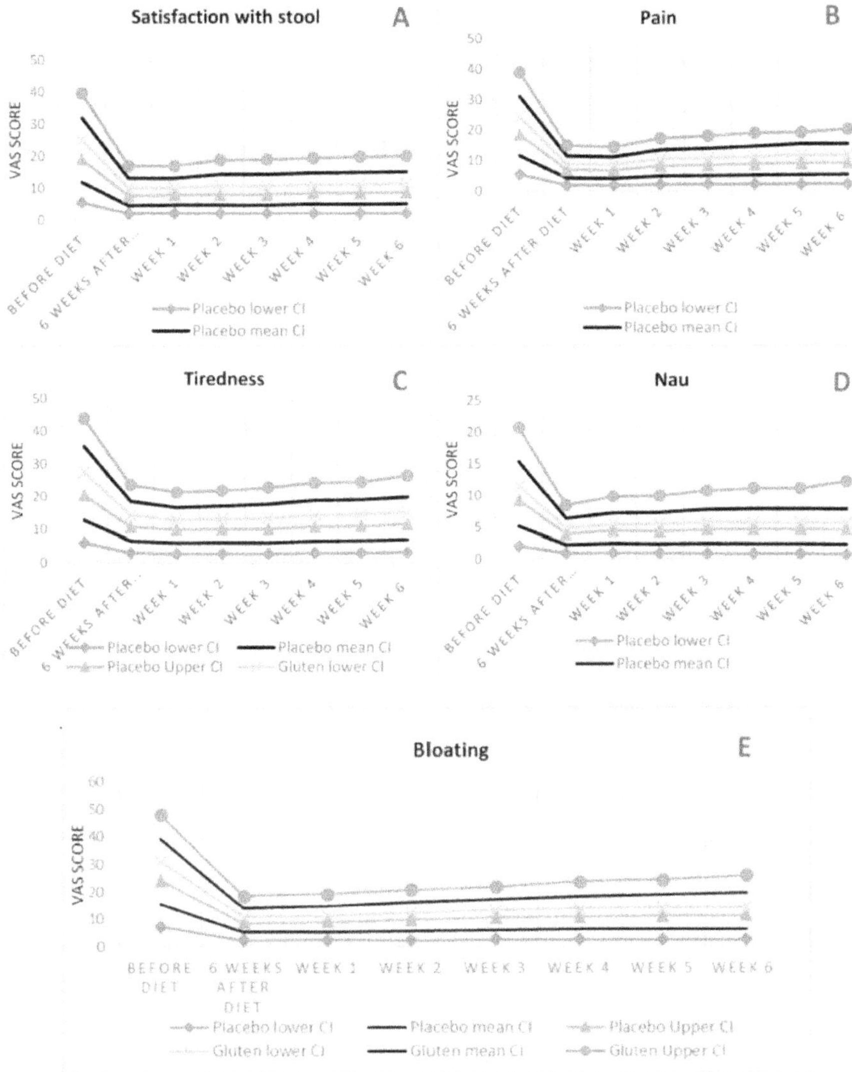



## Fiber

*Bran and insoluble fiber are probably not effective in any form of IBS.*

*Ispaghula (psyllium) and linseed, which are soluble fibers, are probably effective. Linseed seems like it's probably better. It's hard to tell because the studies aren't very good.*

*All studies were done over a max of 1-3 months.*

Sci-Hub | The Effect of Fiber Supplementation on Irritable Bowel Syndrome: A Systematic Review and Meta-analysis | 10.1038/ajg.2014.195 (scihubtw.tw)

*This meta analysis has a nice risk ratio graph, which is helpful for us. Note that all the results for bran span both sides of the line, so it's unclear whether it works.*

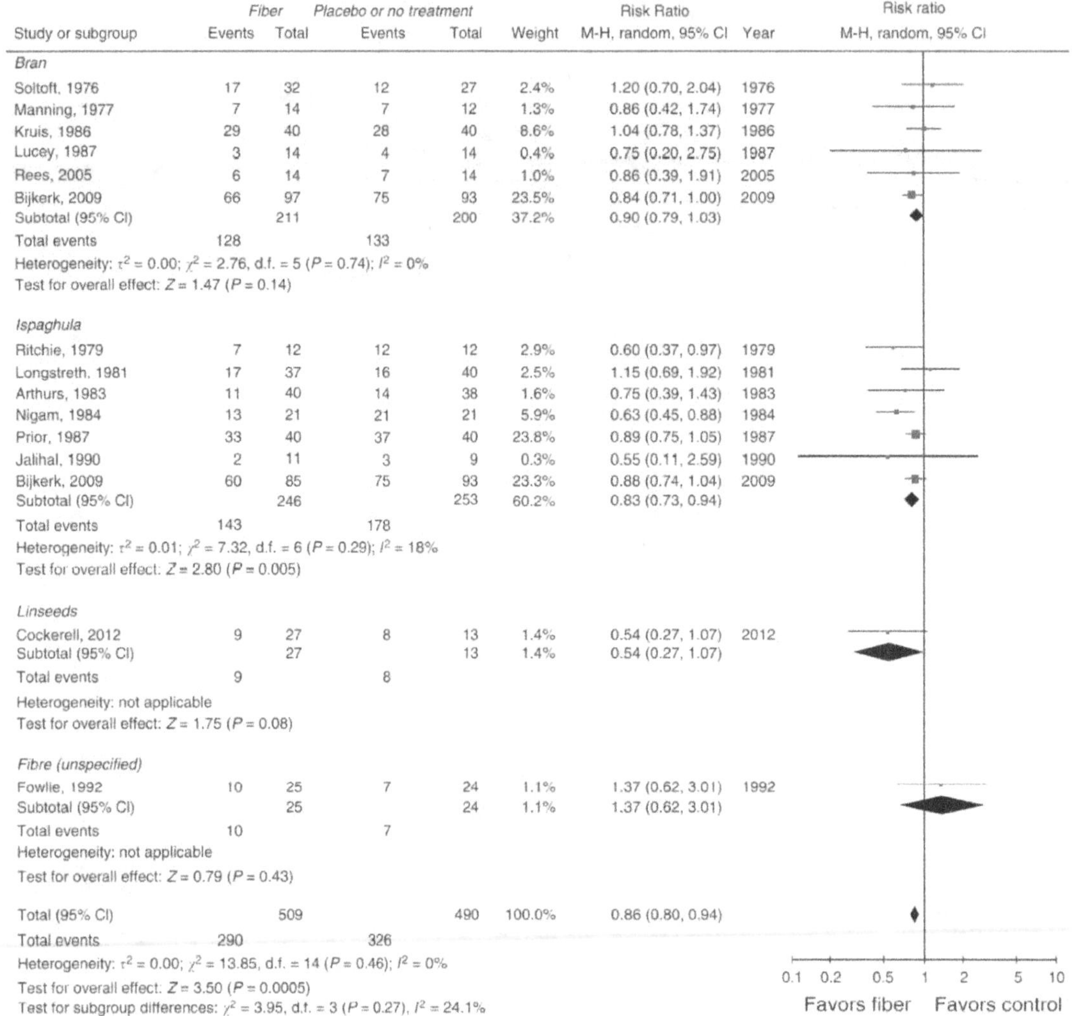

## Anti spasmodics (dicylomine, peppermint oil, pinaverium, trimebutine)

*They have ok effects for abdominal pain and bigger effects for overall symptom scores.*

Bulking agents, antispasmodics and antidepressants for the treatment of irritable bowel syndrome - Ruepert, L - 2011 | Cochrane Library

*This is a Cochrane review paper. Cochrane is usually seen as the gold standard for reviews, although they're often too strict.*

*Also, note that they reverse RR, so RR above 1 is good.*

There was a beneficial effect for antispasmodics over placebo for improvement of abdominal pain (58% of antispasmodic patients improved compared to 46% of placebo; 13 studies; 1392 patients; RR 1.32; 95% CI 1.12 to 1.55; P < 0.001; NNT = 7), global assessment (57% of antispasmodic patients improved compared to 39% of placebo; 22 studies; 1983 patients; RR 1.49; 95% CI 1.25 to 1.77; P < 0.0001; NNT = 5) and symptom score (37% of antispasmodic patients improved compared to 22% of placebo; 4 studies; 586 patients; RR 1.86; 95% CI 1.26 to 2.76; P < 0.01; NNT = 3). Subgroup analyses for different types of antispasmodics found statistically significant benefits for cimteropium/ dicyclomine, peppermint oil, pinaverium and trimebutine. Separate analysis of the studies with adequate allocation concealment found a significant benefit for improvement of abdominal pain.

**Table 2.** Antispasmodics: main results   Open in table viewer

|  | Dichotomous outcomes | Continuous outcomes |
|---|---|---|
|  | RR (95% CI) | SMD (95% CI) |
| Abdominal pain | 1.32 (1.12 to 1.55) | 1.14 (0.47 to 1.81) |
| Global assessment | 1.49 (1.25 to 1.77) |  |
| Symptom score | 1.86 (1.26 to 2.76) | 2.39 (0.50 to 4.29) |

Peppermint oil (Mintoil®) in the treatment of irritable bowel syndrome: A prospective double blind placebo-controlled randomized trial - ScienceDirect

*I wanted to look at peppermint oil specifically because that's what I used to use. It works well according to this study, although note that there's a rebound between 4 to 8 weeks.*

Fifty-seven patients with irritable bowel syndrome according to the Rome II criteria, with normal lactose and lactulose breath tests and negative antibody screening for celiac disease, were treated with peppermint oil (two enteric-coated capsules twice per day or placebo) for 4 weeks in a double blind study. The symptoms were assessed before therapy (T0), after the first 4 weeks of therapy (T4) and 4 weeks after the end of therapy (T8).

At T4, 75% of the patients in the peppermint oil group showed a >50% reduction of basal (T0) total irritable bowel syndrome symptoms score compared with 38% in the placebo group (P < 0.009). With peppermint oil at T4 and at T8 compared with T0 a statistically significant reduction of the total irritable bowel syndrome symptoms score was found (T0: 2.19 ± 0.13, T4: 1.07 ± 0.10*, T8: 1.60 ± 0.10*, *P < 0.01 compared with T0, mean ± S.E.M.), while no change was found with the placebo.

Efficacy of peppermint oil in the treatment of irritable bowel syndrome: a randomized, controlled trial - Gazzetta Medica Italiana Archivio per le Scienze Mediche 2005 April;164(2):119-26 - Minerva Medica - Journals

*Another study showing an effect of peppermint oil, but I wonder if there was a rebound here, too.*

We enrolled 178 consecutive patients affected by IBS, according to the Rome II diagnostic criteria. They were randomized by computer-generated lists to receive either Mintoil 2 capsules t.i.d. before meals for 3 months, or a placebo. A validated questionnaire was administered every 3 weeks to measure the outcome. Data were analysed by $\chi2$ test.

Results. Ninety-one patients (22 M, 69 F; mean age 41 yrs; range 18-72 yrs) received Mintoil, and 87 patients (23 M, 64 F; mean age 44 yrs; range 21-74 yrs) assumed the placebo. Three patients withdrew from the study because of non IBS-related diseases, and two patients because of pyrosis. No other adverse events were recorded.

Peppermint oil, compared to placebo, improved IBS overall symptoms in 73/91 (80%) vs 31/87 (36%) patients (p<0.02). Particularly, significant improvements were achieved for gastroenteric symptoms, in 88/91 (97%) vs 29/87 (33%) patients (p<0.01), psychical discomfort, in 34/91 (37%) vs 16/87 (18%) patients (p<0.05), and socio-familiar impact, in 69/91 (76%) vs 37/87 (43%) patients (p<0.04).

## Discontinuation of proton pump inhibitors

*This isn't really an IBS one, but PPIs do lead to SIBO. Discontinuing them may help.*

Effects of long-term PPI treatment on producing bowel symptoms and SIBO - Compare - 2011 - European Journal of Clinical Investigation - Wiley Online Library

*I only really wanted one study for this, because it's pretty well known, but here you go. They gave patients PPI and accidentally gave them IBS. The other patients who weren't given PPI didn't get IBS.*

Methods Patients with NERD (acid reflux) not complaining of bowel symptoms were selected by upper endoscopy, 24-h pH-metry and a structured questionnaire concerning severity and frequency of bloating, flatulence, abdominal pain, diarrhoea and constipation. Patients were treated with esomeprazole 20 mg bid for 6 months. Prior to and after 8 weeks and 6 months of therapy, patients received the structured questionnaire and underwent evaluation of SIBO by glucose hydrogen breath test (GHBT).

Results Forty-two patients with NERD were selected out of 554 eligible patients. After 8 weeks of PPI treatment, patients complained of bloating, flatulence, abdominal pain and diarrhoea in 43%, 17%, 7% and 2%, respectively. After 6 months, the incidence of bowel symptoms further increased and GHBT (glucose hydrogen breath test) was found positive in 11/42 (26%) patients. By a post hoc analysis, a significant ($P < 0.05$) percentage of patients (8/42) met Rome III criteria for irritable bowel syndrome.

## Antidepressants

*Antidepressants probably make you feel better if you have IBS, in the same way that therapy would. They don't have any other effects.*

Paroxetine to Treat Irritable Bowel Syndrome Not Responding... : Official journal of the American College of Gastroenterology | ACG (lww.com)

*Note that well-being improves with paroxetine, which is an antidepressant, but specific IBS related symptoms do not.*

In Group 2, overall well-being improved more with paroxetine than with placebo (63.3%vs 26.3%; p = 0.01), but abdominal pain, bloating, and social functioning did not. With paroxetine, food avoidance decreased (p = 0.03) and work functioning was marginally better (p = 0.08). Before unblinding, more paroxetine recipients than placebo recipients wanted to continue their study medication (84%vs 37%; p < 0.001).

The Effect of Trimipramine in Patients with the Irritable Bowel Syndrome: A Double-Blind Study: Scandinavian Journal of Gastroenterology: Vol 17, No 7 (tandfonline.com)

*This one shows that trimipramine helps when given a bedtime, for both IBS scores and quality of life. However, I'm not entirely sure what this study is measuring, because there's a lot of vomiting in this study. IBS patients shouldn't be vomiting this much.*

 61 patients were given either 50 mg trimipramine at bedtime or identically looking coded placebo in a prospective study for 4 weeks. The complaints were graded on an analogue scale by both the patients and the physicians. The results showed that the complaint scores were significantly reduced to about half in the placebo group. In the group treated with trimipramine a significantly greater reduction was found for the scores of vomiting, sleeplessness, depression, and for the mucus content of stools. The scores for tiredness during treatment had decreased less in the group receiving trimipramine than in the one receiving placebo. These improvements occurred already during the first week of treatment.

## Table IV. Number of stools per day, mean (ranges)

| Treatment | No. of patients | No. of stools | |
| --- | --- | --- | --- |
| | | Before | After |
| Placebo | 31 | 2.6 (0–5) | 2.0 (0–4) |
| Trimipramine | 30 | 2.4 (0–5) | 1.6 (0-3) |

Cognitive-behavioral therapy versus education and desipramine versus placebo for moderate to severe functional bowel disorders - ScienceDirect

*This is a fun study which compared therapy vs. desipramine, which is an antidepressant. Therapy came out better than desipramine, desipramine came out kind of better than placebo but it's hard to tell. This one breaks out the "intention to treat" vs. "per protocol", which basically means that there were a lot of patients who they intended to treat but didn't (i.e. they dropped out). Also, if you read between the lines, this sort of detailed "subgroup analysis", where they try to get really specific about who would benefit from desipramine, is usually an attempt to rescue a study that went poorly so they have to find some benefit somewhere. Not a good study!*

The intention-to-treat analysis showed CBT as significantly more effective than EDU ($P$ = 0.0001; responder rate, 70% CBT vs. 37% EDU; number needed to treat [NNT ], 3.1). DES did not show significant benefit over PLA in the intention-to-treat analysis ($P$ = 0.16; responder rate, 60% DES vs. 47% PLA; NNT, 8.1) but did show a statistically significant benefit in the per-protocol analysis ($P$ = 0.01; responder rate, 73% DES vs. 49% PLA; NNT, 5.2), especially when participants with nondetectable blood levels of DES were excluded ($P = 0.002$). Improvement was best gauged by satisfaction with treatment. Subgroup analyses showed that DES was beneficial over PLA for moderate more than severe symptoms, abuse history, no depression, and diarrhea-predominant symptoms;

Clinical trial: the effect of amitriptyline in patients with diarrhoea-predominant irritable bowel syndrome - VAHEDI - 2008 - Alimentary Pharmacology & Therapeutics - Wiley Online Library

*This study seems to have a strong effect for low dose amitriptyline, and was overall a well performed study.*

Patients were randomly assigned to receive either 10 mg amitriptyline daily or placebo. Subjects were followed up for 2 months and symptoms were assessed using a questionnaire.

Patients receiving amitriptyline showed greater complete response, defined as loss of all symptoms, compared with those receiving placebo (68% vs. 28%, $P = 0.01$).

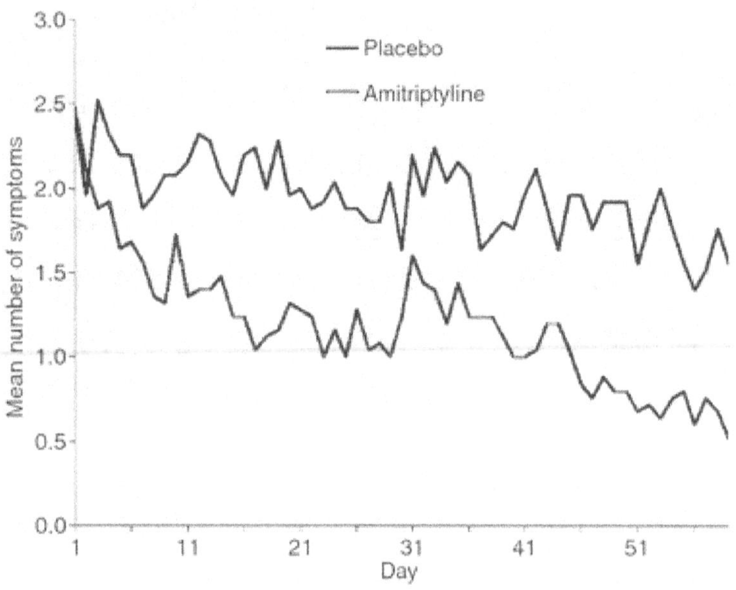


A randomized controlled trial of imipramine in patients with irritable bowel syndrome (nih.gov)

*This study has a remarkably high dropout rate, and it's hard to even know what to think. Why did half the study leave?*

One hundred and seven patients were enrolled by advertisement or referral by general practitioners and 56 (31 imipramine: 25 placebo) completed the 16-wk study. Baseline characteristics were comparable. A high overall dropout rate was noted in the imipramine and placebo arms (47.5% *vs* 47.9%, $P > 0.05$), a mean of 25.0 and 37.4 d from enrollment, respectively ($P < 0.05$). At the end of 12 wk, there was a significant difference in global symptom relief with imipramine over placebo (per-protocol: 80.6% *vs* 48.0%, $P = 0.01$) and a trend on intent-to-treat (ITT) analysis (42.4% *vs* 25.0%, $P = 0.06$). This improvement was evident early and persisted to week 16 ($P = 0.024$ and $0.053$ by per-protocol and ITT analyses, respectively).

*This study compared psychotherapy vs. paroxetine vs. routine care. Psychotherapy actually came out on top.*

Seventy-two patients with IBS participated in a 12-week, double-blind, randomized, placebo-controlled study of paroxetine-CR (12.5 mg–50 mg/day).

In intent-to-treat analyses, there were no significant differences between paroxetine-CR (N = 36) and placebo (N = 36) on reduction in Composite Pain Scores, although the proportion of responders on CGI–I was significantly higher in the paroxetine-CR group.

Patients with severe IBS were randomly allocated to receive 8 sessions of individual psychotherapy, 20 mg daily of the specific serotonin reuptake inhibitor (SSRI) antidepressant, paroxetine, or routine care by a gastroenterologist and general practitioner.

Both psychotherapy and paroxetine were superior to treatment as usual in improving the

physical aspects of health-related quality of life (SF-36 physical component score improvement,

5.2 [SEM, 1.26], 5.8 [SEM, 1.0], and −0.3 [SEM, 1.17]; $P < 0.001$), but there was no difference in the psychological component. During the follow-up year, psychotherapy but not paroxetine was associated with a significant reduction in health care costs compared with treatment as usual (psychotherapy, $976 [SD, $984]; paroxetine, $1252 [SD, $1616]; and treatment as usual, $1663 [SD, $3177]).



*This study weirdly looked at rectal sensitivity as a measure, as well as pain. It showed fluoxetine helped with pain, but not with any IBS specific measures.*

Forty non-depressed IBS patients underwent a rectal barostat study to assess the sensitivity to rectal distention before and after 6 weeks of treatment with fluoxetine 20 mg or placebo. Abdominal pain scores, individual gastrointestinal symptoms, global symptom relief, and psychologic symptoms were assessed before and after the intervention

Fluoxetine did not significantly alter the threshold for discomfort/pain relative to placebo, either in hypersensitive (19 ± 3 vs. 22 ± 2 mm Hg above MDP) or in normosensitive (34 ± 2 vs. 39 ± 4 mm Hg above MDP) IBS patients. Overall, 53% of fluoxetine-treated patients and 76% of placebo-treated patients reported significant abdominal pain scores after 6 weeks (not significant). In contrast, in hypersensitive patients only, fluoxetine significantly reduced the number of patients reporting significant abdominal pain. Gastrointestinal symptoms, global symptom relief, and psychologic symptoms were not altered.



*This study found an effect of citalopram on pain and bloating, but not really on IBS specific measures.*

Twenty three non-depressed IBS patients were recruited from a tertiary care centre and included in a crossover trial comparing six weeks of treatment with the SSRI citalopram (20 mg for three weeks, 40 mg for three weeks) with placebo. IBS symptom severity was the primary outcome measure, and depression and anxiety scores were also measured.

After three and six weeks of treatment, citalopram significantly improved abdominal pain, bloating, impact of symptoms on daily life, and overall well being compared with placebo. There was only a modest effect on stool pattern.

Citalopram Provides Little or No Benefit in Nondepressed Patients With Irritable Bowel Syndrome - ScienceDirect

*This study found no effect of citalopram.*

Patients from primary, secondary, and tertiary care settings were randomly assigned to receive citalopram (20 mg/day for 4 weeks, then 40 mg/day for 4 weeks) or placebo in a study with double-masking and concealed allocation. Symptoms were assessed weekly, and IBS-QOL and rectal sensation by barostat were assessed at the beginning and end of the study.

The effect of fluoxetine in patients with pain and constipation-predominant irritable bowel syndrome: a double-blind randomized-controlled study - VAHEDI - 2005 - Alimentary Pharmacology & Therapeutics - Wiley Online Library

*This study found a big effect of fluoxetine on constipation, and seemed well-performed. They didn't check if their patients were anxious or depressed, though.*

Fluoxetine was significantly more effective than placebo in decreasing abdominal discomfort, relieving feeling and sense of bloating, increasing frequency of bowel movements and decreasing consistency of stool. Mean number of symptoms per patient decreased from 4.6 to 0.7 in the fluoxetine group vs. 4.5 to 2.9 in controls ($P < 0.001$).

Talley: Antidepressant therapy (imipramine and citalopram... - Google Scholar

*This study didn't find any effect for citalopram, but it did find it for imipramine.*

Of 51 IBS patients randomized, baseline characteristics were comparable among the treatment arms; themajority was diarrhea-predominant. Adequate relief of IBS symptoms (primary endpoint) was similar for each treat-ment arm. Improvements in bowel symptom severity rating for interference (P= 0.05) and distress (P= 0.02) were greater with imipramine versus placebo, but improvements in abdominal pain were not. There was a greater improvement in depression score (P = 0.08) and in the SF-36 Mental Component Score (P= 0.07), with imipramine. Citalopram was not superior to placebo. Approximately 20% of the variance in scores was explained by treatment differences for abdominal pain, bowel symptom severity disability, depression and the mental component of the SF-36.

**Rifaximin**

*Rifaximin can definitely benefit IBS-D, and may help IBS-C. It doesn't seem to have any side effects.*

Rifaximin for Irritable Bowel Syndrome (nih.gov)

*This is a metastudy of the 4 studies they found that tested rifaximin. Rifaximin came out pretty well.*

| Source | Dosage | Control | IBS Type | Diagnosis Criteria | Randomization | Blinding | Allocation Concealed |
|---|---|---|---|---|---|---|---|
| Sharara et al 2006 | 400 mg bid | Placebo | Diarrhea, constipation, mixed types | Rome II | Yes | Yes | Yes |
| Pimentel et al 2006 | 400 mg tid | Placebo | Not defined | Rome I | Yes | Yes | No |
| Lembo et al 2008 | 550 mg bid | Placebo | With diarrhea | Rome II | Yes | Yes | No |
| Pimentel et al 2011 | 550 mg tid | Placebo | Without constipation | Rome II | Yes | Yes | Yes |

IBS = irritable bowel syndrome.

| Study or Subgroup | rifaximin Events | rifaximin Total | Placebo Events | Placebo Total | Weight | Risk Ratio M-H, Fixed, 95% CI |
|---|---|---|---|---|---|---|
| Lembo 2008 | 62 | 191 | 41 | 197 | 18.2% | 1.56 [1.11, 2.19] |
| Pimentel 2006 | 16 | 43 | 9 | 44 | 4.0% | 1.82 [0.90, 3.66] |
| Pimentel2011 | 212 | 624 | 171 | 634 | 76.4% | 1.26 [1.06, 1.49] |
| Sharara 2006 | 10 | 37 | 3 | 33 | 1.4% | 2.97 [0.89, 9.89] |
| **Total (95% CI)** | | 895 | | 908 | 100.0% | 1.36 [1.18, 1.58] |
| Total events | 300 | | 224 | | | |

Heterogeneity: Chi$^2$ = 3.71, df = 3 (P = 0.29); I$^2$ = 19%
Test for overall effect: Z = 4.13 (P < 0.0001)

Favours placebo    Favours rifaximin

## Abdominal Pain

No significant heterogeneity in the occurrence of abdominal pain during the treatment period was observed between the 3 RCTs in which abdominal pain was reported (I2=0%).

## Nausea

No significant heterogeneity in the occurrence of nausea during the treatment period was observed between the 3 RCTs in which nausea was reported (I2=0%).

## Vomiting

No significant heterogeneity in the occurrence of vomiting during the treatment period was observed between the 3 RCTs in which vomiting was reported (I2=0%)

## Headache

No significant heterogeneity in the occurrence of headache during the treatment period was observed between the 3 RCTs in which headache was reported (I2=0%).

## Vitamin D

*Very high doses of vitamin D every 2 weeks probably improve IBS symptoms.*

Effect of vitamin D on gastrointestinal symptoms and health-related quality of life in irritable bowel syndrome patients: a randomized double-blind clinical trial - Abbasnezhad - 2016 - Neurogastroenterology & Motility - Wiley Online Library

*I like this one because it's actually long term. It shows remarkably big effects, too.*

A total of 90 IBS patients participated in this double-blind, randomized, placebo-controlled study. Participants were randomly selected to receive either 50 000 IU vitamin D3 or a placebo fortnightly for a period of 6 months. Patients reported their IBS symptoms at the baseline and monthly during intervention periods

Over the 6-month intervention period, a significantly greater improvement in IBS symptoms such as abdominal pain and distention, flatulence, rumbling, and overall gastrointestinal (GI) symptoms (except dissatisfaction with bowel habits) was observed in the patients receiving vitamin D as compared to the placebo group. The IBSSS and the IBS-QoL scores in the vitamin D group significantly improved compared to the placebo group postintervention (mean IBSSS score change: −53.82 ± 23.3 *vs* −16.85 ± 25.01, *p* < 0.001, respectively; mean IBS-QoL score change: 14.26 ± 3 *vs* 11 ± 2.34, *p* < 0.001, respectively).

Co-Administration of Soy Isoflavones and Vitamin D in Management of Irritable Bowel Disease (plos.org)

*This one also tests isoflavones, and seems to find a bigger effect of soy isoflavones than vitamin D, although both have an effect. It was only for 6 weeks, though. Also, the groups seem really poorly assigned: the before scores are all over the place.*

In a factorial blinded randomized clinical trial, 100 women with IBS (age:18-75yr, were randomly assigned in 4 arms to receive either placebo of vitamin D and placebo of soy isoflavones (P+P), or placebo of vitamin D and soy isoflavones (P+S), or vitamin D and placebo of soy isoflavones (D+P), or vitamin D and soy isoflavones (D+S) for 6 weeks. Dosage of soy isoflavone was 2 capsules of 20 mg soy isoflavones per day, and dosage of vitamin D was one pearl of 50'000 IU biweekly. The clinical outcomes were IBS symptoms severity scores (IBS-SSS), disease-specific quality of life (IBS-QOL) and total score (IBS-TS) that evaluated at weeks 0, 6, and 10, and compared to each other.

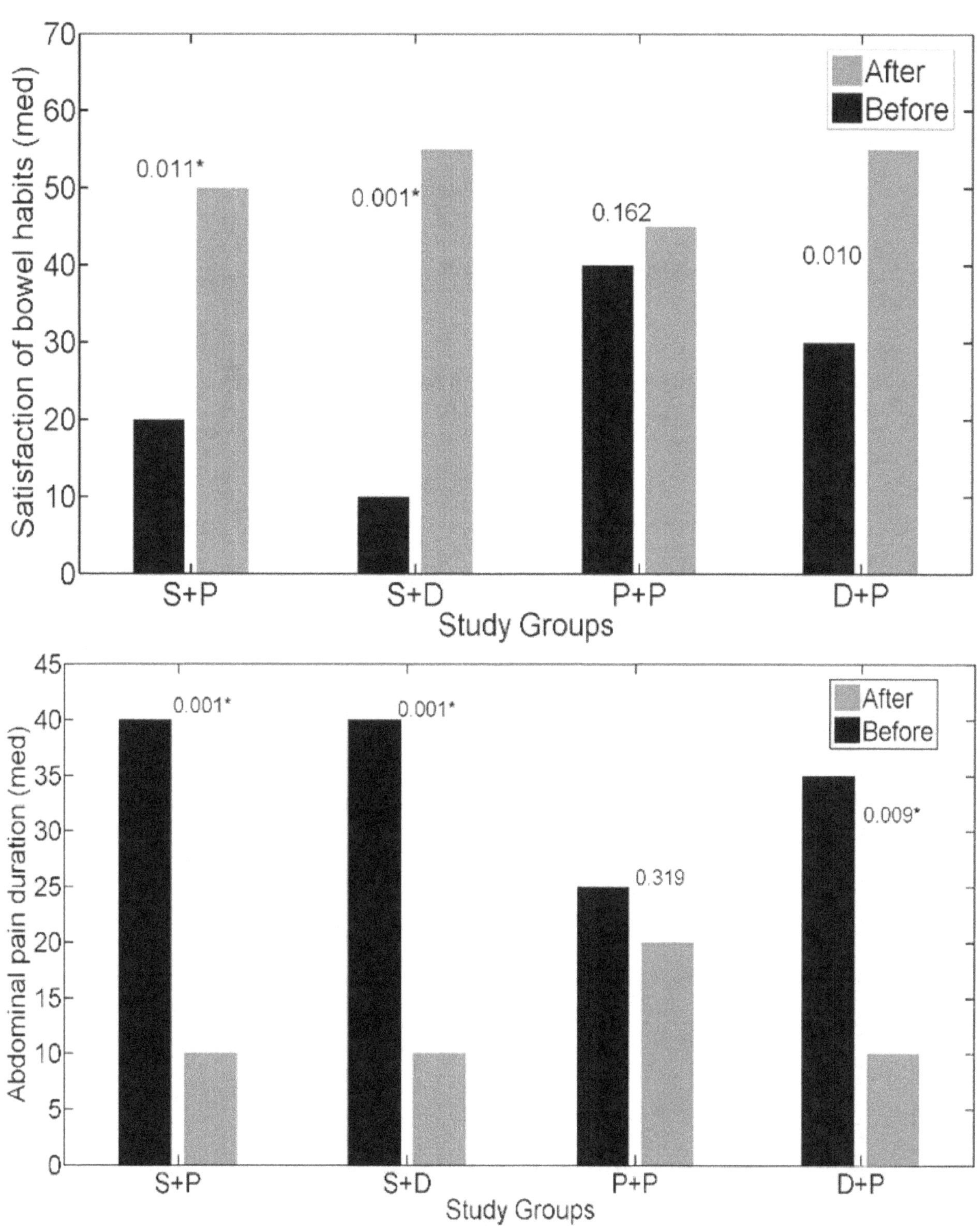


**Soy isoflavones**

*Soy isoflavones may improve IBS, but it's hard to tell.*

*This is just testing soy isoflavones. It's really hard to tell what's going on here, as either the soy isoflavones did show some amount of improvement that was almost significant (p value of 0.068), or they actually made things worse.*

In a randomized double blind placebo-controlled clinical trial, 67 patients with IBS were allocated to consume either soy isoflavones capsules or a placebo for 6 weeks. The primary outcome was a significant reduction in symptoms severity score and the secondary outcome was a significant improvement in quality of life.

45 participants completed the study. There was no significant changes in mean differences of symptoms severity score between the two groups; however soy isoflavone supplementation could significantly improve the quality of life scores (*p*=0.009).

Table 3

**The mean difference of the effect of soy isoflavones versus placebo on SSS, IBS-QOL and total score between the two groups**

| Characteristic | Soy (n=22) | | Placebo (n=23) | | Crude p-value | Adjusted p-value | $R^2$ |
|---|---|---|---|---|---|---|---|
| | Crude | Adjusted | Crude | Adjusted | | | |
| SSS, Mean (SE) | 12.77(1.74) | 13.36(2.09) | 19.74(2.52) | 19.18(2.04) | 0.029 | 0.068 | 0.371 |
| IBS-QOL, Mean(SE) | 41.68 (6.07) | 33.34(4.63) | 44.17(6.98) | 52.15(4.52) | 0.789 | 0.009 | 0.607 |
| Total score, Mean(SE) | 69.76 (5.39) | 68.97(3.88) | 26.30(3.30) | 27.03(3.68) | <0.001 | <0.001 | 0.734 |

Notes: Crude Significances are based on independent t test and adjusted significances are based on ANCOVA with factors age, BMI, IQB (IBS- QOL baseline) and before baseline value of each factor as covariates. SSS: Severity scoring system. IBS- QOL: Inflammatory bowel syndrome-Quality of life

## Acupuncture

*Acupuncture probably doesn't work better than fake acupuncture.*



*This one seems self-explanatory. Also, I'm biased against acupuncture.*

We found no evidence of an improvement with acupuncture relative to sham (placebo) acupuncture for symptom severity (SMD-0.11, 95%CI −0.35 to 0.13; 4 RCTs; 281 patients) or quality of life (SMD = −0.03, 95%CI −0.27 to 0.22; 3 RCTs; 253 patients).

## Probiotics

*Probiotics may help a little bit but it's hard to tell. This is compounded by the fact that how probiotics are stored and processed matters a lot to whether they survive all the way to colonize your digestive tract.*

Effect of probiotic species on irritable bowel syndrome symptoms:A bring up to date meta-analysis

*This study only looked at species, and not at formulation. Also, I don't trust that some probiotics improve pain, but not distension. That doesn't make sense.*

**Results:** meta-analysis was performed with 10 of 24 studies identified as suitable for inclusion. Probiotics improved pain scores if they contained *Bifidobacterium breve* (SMD, -0.34; 95% CI, -0.66; -0.02), *Bifidobacterium longum* (SMD, -0.48; 95% CI, -0.91; -0.06), or *Lactobacillus acidophilus* (SMD, -0.31; 95% CI, -0.61; -0.01) species. Distension scores were improved by probiotics containing *B. breve* (SMD, -0.45; 95% CI, -0.77; -0.13), *Bifidobacterium infantis, Lactobacillus casei,* or *Lactobacillus plantarum* (SMD, -0.53; 95% CI, -1.00; -0.06) species. All probiotic species tested improved flatulence: *B. breve* (SMD, -0.42; 95% CI, -0.75;-0.10), *B. infantis, L. casei, L. plantarum* (SMD, -0.60; 95% CI, -1.07; -0.13), *B. longum, L. acidophilus, Lactobacillus bulgaricus, and Streptococcus salivarius ssp. thermophilus* (SMD, -0.61; 95% CI, -1.01; -0.21). There was not a clear positive effect of probiotics concerning the quality of life.

The utility of probiotics in the treatment of irritable bowel syndrome: a systematic review - Database of Abstracts of Reviews of Effects (DARE): Quality-assessed Reviews - NCBI Bookshelf (nih.gov)

*This is a meta study. It discusses that the only properly performed studies that showed a good effect were on B.infantis.*

Sixteen RCTs (n=1,342) met the inclusion criteria. Studies scored between 5 and 12 points on the Rome II methodology scale. Eleven studies were considered to be of suboptimal design (precise definition of suboptimal was not clear).

Two of the appropriately-designed RCTs evaluated Bifidobacterium infantis 35624 and reported statistically significant improvements in abdominal pain/discomfort, bloating/distension and/or bowel movement relative to placebo (p<0.05). In these two trials B. infantis 35624 was given daily for four or eight weeks as 1x1010 live cells in malted milk drink or 1x106, 1x108 or 1x1010 colony forming units per millilitre in capsule form. None of the other studies described as appropriately designed showed significant improvements in IBS symptoms.

No studies reported quantifiable data on relative tolerability or adverse events.



*This is a meta study on B. infantis specifically. They found that single B. infantis didn't help, but combination B. infantis did. That doesn't really make sense to me. I'd bet it's a formulation problem.*

A total of five studies were identified as suitable for inclusion, including three studies with single probiotic B. infantis and two studies with composite probiotics containing B. infantis. Treatment with single probiotic B. infantis didn't impact on abdominal pain, bloating/distention, or bowel habit satisfaction among IBS patients. However, patients who received composite probiotics containing B. infantis had significantly reduced abdominal pain (SMD, 0.22; 95% CI, 0.03–0.41) and bloating/distention (SMD, 0.30; 95% CI, 0.04–0.56). After combining the data from six studies, the improvement of bloating/distention among IBS patients remained significant (SMD, 0.21; 95% CI, 0.07–0.35).

**Mesalazine**

*Mesalazine is probably not effective in IBS.*



*So, this paper basically found that both placebo and mesalazine had the same "response rate", which was 67%. Then they tried to rescue it by doing a bunch of complicated statistics, but it really didn't work that well.*

For the primary endpoint, the responder patients were 68.6% in the mesalazine group versus 67.4% in the placebo group (p=0.870; 95% CI −12.8 to 15.1). In explorative analyses, with the 75% rule or >75% rule, the percentage of responders was greater in the mesalazine group with a difference over placebo of 11.6% (p=0.115; 95% CI −2.7% to 26.0%) and 5.9% (p=0.404; 95% CI −7.8% to 19.4%), respectively, although these differences were not significant. For the key secondary endpoint, overall symptoms improved in the mesalazine group and reached a significant difference of 15.1% versus placebo (p=0.032; 95% CI 1.5% to 28.7%) with the >75% rule.

**Loperamide**

*This study basically showed that loperamide works well.*

Loperamide treatment accelerated gastric emptying, compared with placebo (1.2 +- 0.1 vs 1.5 +- 0.1 hr; P < 0.001) and delayed both small bowel (6.2 + 0.3 vs 4.3 + 0.3 hr; P < 0.001) and whole gut transit (56 +- 5 vs 42 +_ 4 hr; P < 0.01). Eighteen patients said they felt better taking loperamide compared with placebo and, at follow up, 15 of these patients remained satisfied with the effects of the drug. Most symptoms improved significantly on placebo compared with the baseline period, but three of these [diarrhea (P < 0.01), urgency (P < 0.01) and borborygmi (P < 0.05)] showed a further significant improvement on loperamide. Improvement in diarrhea was not associated with any change in stool weight but was associated with reductions in stool frequency (P < 0.001), passage of unformed stools (P < 0.01), and incidence of urgency (P < 0.001).

A Double-Blind Placebo-Controlled Trial with Loperamide in Irritable Bowel Syndrome: Scandinavian Journal of Gastroenterology: Vol 31, No 5 (tandfonline.com)

*Loperamide improved IBS symptoms, but increased pain at night.*

Clinical variables and social and personal relationships were similar for the loperamide group (*n* = 35), the placebo group (*n* = 34), the dropouts (*n* = 21), and the controls. Somatic diseases and mental disturbances were increased in the patients compared with the controls. Throughout the 5 weeks of treatment an improved stool consistency (32%), reduced defecation frequency (36%), and reduced intensity of pain (30%) were found in the loperamide group. An increase in nightly pain was observed in the loperamide group.

Loperamide Treatment of the Irritable Bowel Syndrome: Scandinavian Journal of Gastroenterology: Vol 22, No sup130 (tandfonline.com)

*Loperamide helped diarrhea but made constipation worse (duh).*

In a group of patients with painless diarrhoea (n = 16) there was a highly significant improvement in stool frequency and consistency. In a group with alternating bowel habits and abdominal pain (n = 21) there was also a statistically significant improvement in stool frequency and consistency as well as significantly fewer painful days during loperamide treatment. Patients with alternating bowel habits and no pain (n = 12) experienced no symptomatic improvement, and patients with constipation (n = 9) generally felt worse on loperamide. No side effects were encountered.

Loperamide in Treatment of Irritable Bowel Syndrome—A Double-Blind Placebo Controlled Study: Scandinavian Journal of Gastroenterology: Vol 22, No sup130 (tandfonline.com)

*Loperamide helps diarrhea and diarrhea-related symptoms.*

The effects of loperamide in patients with IBS (all had diarrhoea as a main symptom) were studied in a double-blind placebo controlled trial. Subjective overall response, stool consistency and six individual symptoms (urgency, pain, frequency, flatulence, borborygmi and painful propulsions) were studied over a 13 week long treatment period. Twenty-one patients out of 25 completed the trial, 11 in the loperamide group and 10 in the placebo group. A significant advantage for loperamide was found for stool consistency (p<0.001), pain (p<0.02) and urgency (p<0.05). Subjective overall response was also significantly better in the loperamide group (p<0.03).

## Fecal transplant

*Results vary really widely. Worth a shot if you're desperate.*

Efficacy of Fecal Microbiota Transplantation in Irritable Bowel Syndrome: A Systematic Review and Meta-Analysis (nih.gov)

*This meta analysis threw out half the studies for not being well-performed. The rest are presented below. Note that two of them show a big positive effect, and two of them do not. The two negative ones did capsule, the two positive ones did colonoscopy and nasojejunal tubes.*

| Study | FMT Events | FMT Total | Placebo Events | Placebo Total | Risk Ratio | RR | 95%-CI | Weight |
|---|---|---|---|---|---|---|---|---|
| Johnsen 2017 | 36 | 60 | 12 | 30 | | 1.50 | [0.92; 2.44] | 27.1% |
| Holvoet 2018 | 21 | 42 | 6 | 22 | | 1.83 | [0.87; 3.87] | 22.5% |
| Aroniadis 2018 | 10 | 24 | 15 | 24 | | 0.67 | [0.38; 1.17] | 25.7% |
| Halkjær 2018 | 8 | 26 | 19 | 26 | | 0.42 | [0.23; 0.78] | 24.7% |
| Overall | | 152 | | 102 | | 0.93 | [0.48; 1.79] | 100.0% |
| Total Events | 75 | | 52 | | | | | |

Weights are from random effects analysis
Heterogeneity: $I^2$ = 79%, $\chi^2_3$ = 14.47 ($p < 0.01$)
Clinical Response to FMT: $z$ = −0.22 ($p = 0.83$)

## Antihistamines (especially cromolyn)
*Cromolyn seems to work well in diarrheic IBS.*

Oral Cromolyn Sodium in Comparison with Elimination Diet in the Irritable Bowel Syndrome, Diarrheic Type Multicenter Study of 428 Patients: Scandinavian Journal of Gastroenterology: Vol 30, No 6 (tandfonline.com)

*So, my main problem with this study is that there's zero blinding and no placebo group. They do try to rescue this by showing there's a correlation with response to cromolyn and general allergies, but I'd really like to see a comparison group.*

Symptoms related to the irritable bowel syndrome improved in 60% of patients treated with elimination diet and in 67% of those treated with oral cromolyn sodium (1500 mg/day) for 1 month. Moreover, in both groups clinical results were significantly better in the patients positive to the skin prick test than in the negative ones

Double-blind cross-over trial of oral sodium cromoglycate in patients with irritable bowel syndrome due to food intolerance - LUNARDI - 1991 - Clinical & Experimental Allergy - Wiley Online Library

*This one is double-blinded and placebo controlled, which is nice. It's a small study, which is unfortunate. But they did try very hard to make sure people actually had IBS by ruling out other causes. They also switched the arms to see if people got better or worse when those same patients got switched to cromolyn or placebo. The one thing I don't like is that some poor guy got violent diarrhea on cromolyn, and they just kind of ignored him.*

Patients were allowed to eat the offending foods during the study. Eighteen patients completed the study. Analysis of patients' diary card scores showed a statistically significant difference in favour of sodium cromoglycate. There was a long carry-over effect in the active-placebo order group.

## Miralax (polyethylene glycol)
*Unsurprisingly, Miralax works well.*


*Pretty straightforward Cochrane review finds Miralax does better than Lactulose.*
The findings of our work indicate that Polyethylene glycol is better than lactulose in outcomes of stool frequency per week, form of stool, relief of abdominal pain and the need for additional products. On subgroup analysis, this is seen in both adults and children, except for relief of abdominal pain. Polyethylene Glycol should be used in preference to Lactulose in the treatment of Chronic Constipation.


*This is just a collection of case reports. Nothing too exciting, but Miralax is pretty safe.*
The most common clinical adverse effect was excessively loose or frequent stools that resolved with reduction of the PEG dose. Other adverse effects were minimal and acceptable. Polyethylene glycol does not ferment by colonic bacterial flora and, therefore, does not cause excessive gas production that leads to flatulence or bloating

## Magnesium Citrate powder
*Unsurprisingly, magnesium citrate works well. Unfortunately, it has bad effects.*


*So, there are no good studies on adverse effects of magnesium citrate, mainly because it'd be unethical to do a study to see how sick people got. There are a lot of anecdotes, though, and it doesn't seem worth it to look into it more deeply.*

Many reports indicate that overdose or repetitive ingestion of magnesium-containing cathartics can cause hypermagnesemia, which can be fatal, even in patients with normal renal function. The diagnosis of hypermagnesemia should be considered in patients who present with symptoms of hyporeflexia, lethargy, refractory hypotension, shock, prolonged QT interval, or respiratory depression, and they need immediate attention

## Lactulose
*Worse than magnesium citrate, just relying on the same stuff from above.*

## Bisacodyl
*Again, bisacodyl works well, which is no surprise. It makes people poop.*

*This study seems almost unnecessary. Bisacodyl makes people poop. It can make people poop too much. Some people get unhappy with that.*
Overall satisfaction scores for bowel habits, bothersomeness of constipation, and abdominal discomfort and bloating improved with bisacodyl compared with placebo (unpublished data, see

Table 2). Over the study period, the most common AEs in patients treated with bisacodyl were diarrhea and abdominal pain, experienced by 53.4% and 24.7% of patients, respectively, compared with 1.7% and 2.5% in the placebo group, respectively. 17.8% of the bisacodyl-treated patients withdrew prematurely because of AEs, compared with only 5.0% of the placebo group

Long-term Use of Bisacodyl in Pediatric Functional Constipat... : Journal of Pediatric Gastroenterology and Nutrition (lww.com)
*On the other hand, this is a study showing long term use. Only half of the longterm kids successfully got off bisacodyl, which is not a great response.*
At long-term follow-up 55% of patients were successfully weaned off bisacodyl (median time of 18 months)


**Senna / Sennosides**
*Senna makes people poop violently. That's what it does. All of its positive effects and all of its negative effects can be ascribed to that.*


Are Senna based laxatives safe when used as long term treatment for constipation in children? - ScienceDirect
*Yup, it makes them poop violently. This can cause butthole blisters and pooping at night.*
Eight articles in the literature reported perineal blisters after administration of Senna laxatives in 28 patients. Of those occurrences, 18 patients (64%) had accidental administration of Senna and 10 (36%) had Senna prescribed as a long term treatment. All of the blistering episodes were related to high dose, night-time accidents, or intense diarrhea with a long period of stool to skin contact. At our institution, from 2014 to 2017, we prescribed Senna and have recorded data to 640 patients. During the study period, 17 patients (2.2%) developed blisters during their treatment. Patients who developed blisters had higher doses 60 mg/day; 60 [12–100] vs. 17.5 [1.7–150] (p < 0.001).


Senna Versus Magnesium Oxide for the Treatment of Chronic Co... : Official journal of the American College of Gastroenterology | ACG (lww.com)
*This is comparing senna vs. magnesium. I'm not sure why they used magnesium here instead of polyethylene glycol. Both of them made people poop.*
Ninety patients (mean age, 42 years; 93% women; mean duration of symptoms, 9.9 years) were enrolled; all completed the study. The response rate for overall improvement was 11.7% in the placebo group, 69.2% in the senna group, and 68.3% in the MgO group (P < 0.0001).


**Amitiza (lubiprostone, prescription):**
*Amitiza also makes people poop, and has many of the same effects of other laxatives.*
https://link.springer.com/content/pdf/10.1007/s10620-009-1068-x.pdf#page=1


Lubiprostone-treated patients experienced greater mean numbers of SBMs at week 1 compared with placebo(5.89 versus 3.99,P=0.0001), with significantly greater percentages having SBMs within 24 h of the first dose(61.3% versus 31.4%,P\0.0001).


Adverse effects: nausea, abdominal pain, diarrhea.

**Linaclotide (Linzess , prescription, "Constella" in Canada)**
*Linaclotide makes people poop, but it actually doesn't seem to work that well compared to other laxatives. I'm not sure what the advantage of it would be.*
Linaclotide (Linzess) for Irritable Bowel syndrome With Constipation and For Chronic Idiopathic Constipation (nih.gov)
In all, 804 patients (mean age=44 years, female=90%, white=78%) were evaluated; 33.7% of linaclotide-treated patients were FDA end point responders, vs. 13.9% of placebo-treated patients (P<0.0001) (number needed to treat=5.1, 95% confidence interval (CI): 3.9, 7.1). The pain responder criterion of the FDA end point was met by 48.9% of linaclotide-treated patients vs. 34.5% of placebo-treated patients (number needed to treat=7.0, 95% CI: 4.7, 13.1), and the CSBM responder criterion was met by 47.6% of linaclotide-treated patients, vs. 22.6% of placebo patients (number needed to treat=4.0, 95% CI: 3.2, 5.4). Remaining primary end points (P<0.0001) and all secondary end points (P<0.001), including abdominal pain, abdominal bloating, and bowel symptoms (SBM and CSBM rates, Bristol Stool Form Scale (BSFS) score, and straining), were also statistically significantly improved with linaclotide vs. placebo.

Diarrhea is a very common side effect

**Motegrity (prucalopride, prescription):**
*Motegrity also makes people poop, but doesn't seem to work that well compared to other laxatives. I also don't get the market for this one.*
Prucalopride: safety, efficacy and potential applications
The primary endpoint, in each study, was the proportion of patients passing at least three SCBMs per week during the 12 weeks of the trial, based on an intention-to-treat analysis. All three trials (which assessed 620, 641, and 713 patients, respectively) demonstrated a significant increase in the proportion of patients achieving at least three SCBMs per week compared with placebo. Response rates ranged from 19.5% to 31% with 2 mg prucalopride, 24% to 28% with 4 mg prucalopride, and 9.6% to 12% with placebo.

It's too early to assess its potential usefulness in disorders such as gastroparesis, intestinal pseudo-obstruction, functional dyspepsia and, most importantly, IBS-C.

The most common treatment-associated adverse events were headache (25–30% prucalopride; 12–17% placebo), nausea (12–24%; 8–14%), abdominal pain or cramps (16–23%; 11–19%) and diarrhea (12–19%; 3–5%) [Tack et al. 2009; Quigley et al. 2009; Camilleri et al. 2008b].

**Trulance (plecanatide, prescription):**
*Another laxative with pretty meh results. I don't understand why they keep developing these.*
Efficacy, safety, and tolerability of plecanatide in patient... : Official journal of the American College of Gastroenterology | ACG (lww.com)

The percentage of overall responders in Study 1 was 30.2% and 29.5% for plecanatide 3 and 6 mg, respectively, vs. 17.8% placebo (P< 0.001 for each dose vs. placebo), and in Study 2 was 21.5% (P= 0.009) and 24.0% (P< 0.001) for plecanatide 3 and 6 mg, respectively, compared to 14.2% for placebo. The percentage of sustained efficacy responders (overall responders plus weekly responders for ≥2 of last 4 weeks of the 12-week treatment period) was significantly greater for both doses of plecanatide vs. placebo across both studies

The most common AE was diarrhea (3 mg, 4.3%; 6 mg, 4.0%; placebo, 1.0%). Discontinuation due to diarrhea was infrequent (3 mg, 1.2%; 6 mg, 1.4%; placebo, 0).


**Exercise**

This obviously works. For proof, look at people who take their dogs out to walk before they poop.

**Surgeries**
*The surgeries do what you'd expect: they cut out the parts of the colon that don't work, and stitch the rest back together. A shorter colon means less time to digest and get the water out, so you get diarrhea frequently.*

Surgical Management of Colonic Inertia (nih.gov)
*This isn't super scientific. It's just a survey of results. Overall, people seem to be pretty happy long term with their surgery, or at least that's what they tell doctors who call them up on the phone.*
FitzHarris and colleagues surveyed 75 patients who had undergone TAC IRA a mean of 3.9 years (range 0.5 to 9.6) prior to the survey.14 Using a 54-item validated questionnaire (Gastrointestinal Quality-of-Life Index), the authors found 81% of the patients were at least somewhat pleased with their bowel frequency, but 41% cited abdominal pain, 21% incontinence, and 46% diarrhea at least some of the time. However, 93% stated they would undergo subtotal colectomy again if given a second chance.

**Laparoscopic total colectomy**
Laparoscopic total colectomy for colonic inertia: surgical and functional results | SpringerLink
Preoperative Wexner's constipation score was 22.3 (range 19–29 months) pre surgery and at the end of follow-up was 1.8 (range 0–6) (p < 0.01). The medium level of satisfaction was 8 (range 2–10) and only one patient would not recommend surgery to other patients.

# How I came up with my list of diagnoses

*I did less evaluation of the diagnoses, because they're mostly straightforward and less prone to error than treatments. I did look carefully for epidemiology and unique symptoms.*

## Diverticulitis

*Diverticulitis is marked by bloating, constipation or diarrhea, and cramping. Most notable effect is blood in stool. Obesity/lack of exercise is a contributing factor.*

Symptoms & Causes of Diverticular Disease | NIDDK (nih.gov)

Most people with diverticulosis do not have symptoms. If your diverticulosis causes symptoms, they may include

- bloating
- constipation or diarrhea
- cramping or pain in your lower abdomen

In most cases, when you have diverticular bleeding, you will suddenly have a large amount of red or maroon-colored blood in your stool.

Studies have found links between diverticular disease—diverticulosis that causes symptoms or problems such as diverticular bleeding or diverticulitis—and the following factors:

- certain medicines—including nonsteroidal anti-inflammatory drugs (NSAIDs), such as aspirin, and steroids
- lack of exercise
- obesity
- smoking

## Testing for colon cancer:

*Colon cancer is mostly for people over 45. The best indicator is a fecal occult blood test.*

Sci-Hub | Primary colon cancer: ESMO Clinical Practice Guidelines for diagnosis, adjuvant treatment and follow-up | 10.1093/annonc/mdq168 (scihubtw.tw)

About 70% of patients with colon cancer are >65 years of age and the disease is rare under the age of 45 (2 per 100 000/year).

Colorectal cancer most commonly occurs sporadically and is inherited in only 5%–10% of cases. Migrant studies indicate that when populations move from a low-risk area (e.g. Japan) to a high-risk area (e.g. the USA), the incidence increases rapidly within the first generation of migrants.

Smoking has consistently been associated with large colorectal adenomas, which are generally accepted as precursors for cancer. An updated review suggested a temporal pattern consistent with an induction period of three to four decades between genotoxic exposure and the diagnosis of colorectal cancer. In the USA one in five colorectal cancers may be potentially attributable to tobacco use.

Inflammatory bowel diseases (Crohn's disease and ulcerative colitis) increase the risk of colon cancer

Patients who have had previous malignant disease are also at great risk of developing a second colorectal tumour

The metabolic syndrome (high blood pressure, increased waist circumference, hypertriglyceridaemia, low levels of high-density lipoprotein cholesterol or diabetes/ hyperglycaemia) had a modest, positive association with colorectal cancer incidence among men, but not among women

Because early cancer produces no symptoms and because many of the symptoms are non-specific (change in bowel habits, general abdominal discomfort, weight loss with no apparent cause, constant tiredness),

 Up to now two strategies have been available: faecal occult blood test (FOBT) and endoscopy.

Influence of dietary factors on colorectal cancer survival (nih.gov)

Colorectal cancer (CRC) is one of the most common cancers in the Western world. It is widely accepted that environmental factors, especially dietary factors, are involved in the aetiology of CRC. High intakes of fat, red meat, refined sugar, and energy have been associated with an increased risk of CRC

## Inflammatory bowel disease

*IBD is mostly diarrhea, especially bloody diarrhea. If your relatives have IBD, you're more likely to have IBD.*

The Diagnostic Approach to Monogenic Very Early Onset Inflammatory Bowel Disease - ScienceDirect

Twin studies have provided the best evidence for a genetic predisposition to IBD, which is stronger for CD than UC.

Genetic disorders that affect intestinal epithelial barrier function include dystrophic epidermolysis bullosa,32 Kindler syndrome,32 familial diarrhea caused by dominant activating mutations in guanylate cyclase C,33 X-linked ectodermal dysplasia and immunodeficiency,34 and ADAM17 deficiency.35

As high as 40% of patients with chronic granulomatous disease develop CD-like intestinal inflammation.

VEOIBD has been described in a number of hyperinflammatory and autoinflammatory disorders such as mevalonate kinase deficiency,54, 55 phospholipase C-γ2 defects,56 familial Mediterranean fever,57, 58, 59 Hermansky–Pudlak syndrome (type 1, 4, and 6),60, 61, 62, 63, 64 X-linked lymphoproliferative syndrome type 165 and type 2,66, 67, 68 or familial hemophagocytic lymphohistiocytosis type 5

Disorders associated with IBD-like immunopathology include B-cell defects such as common variable immunodeficiency (CVID), hyper-immunoglobulin (Ig) M syndrome, and agammaglobulinemia.75, 76, 77, 78, 79 Several other primary immune deficiencies, such as Wiskott–Aldrich syndrome80 (WAS) and atypical SCID or Omenn syndrome81, 82 can also cause IBD-like intestinal inflammation.

Cow's milk protein allergy is common and can cause severe colitis that resembles UC and even requires hospitalization. It manifests typically within the first 2 to 3 months of exposure to cow's milk protein. This may be apparent with breast-feeding or only after introducing formula feeding. Colitis resolves after cow's milk is removed from the diet, so a trial of exclusive feeding with an amino acid–based infant formula is a customary treatment strategy for all VEOIBD diagnosed when the patient is younger than 1 year of age.

ESPGHAN Revised Porto Criteria for the Diagnosis of Inflamma... : Journal of Pediatric Gastroenterology and Nutrition (lww.com)

Bloody diarrhea is the most common presenting symptom in UC whereas CD may present with vague abdominal pain, diarrhea, unexplained anemia, fever, weight loss, or growth retardation as frequently reported symptoms. The classic "triad" of abdominal pain, diarrhea, and weight loss occurs in only 25% of patients with CD

**Hypothyroidism**

*Hypothyroidism symptoms listed below, with asterisks for the most notable ones.*

Hypothyroidism: an update: South African Family Practice: Vol 54, No 5 (tandfonline.com)

Arthralgias (joint pain)

Cold intolerance*

Constipation

Depression

Difficulty concentrating

Menorrhagia (heavy flow)

Myalgias (muscle pain)

Weakness

Weight gain

Dry skin

Fatigue*

Hair thinning/hair loss

Memory impairment

## Giardiasis

*Giardiasis is via contamination, and usually includes diarrhea.*

Sci-Hub | Giardiasis – why do the symptoms sometimes never stop? | 10.1016/j.pt.2009.11.010 (scihubtw.tw)

Transmission of Giardia is via the faecal–oral route, either indirectly through contaminated water or food, or directly from person to person.

Giardia infection is usually associated with diarrhoea, but can be either asymptomatic or responsible for a broad clinical spectrum, with symptoms ranging from acute to chronic [4]; diarrhoea can occur with or without malabsorption syndrome; there can be nausea, vomiting, and weight loss [5]. Occasionally, Giardia infection can be associated with pruritis and urticaria [6], uveitis [7], sensitisation towards food antigens [8,9] and synovitis [10]. Children might also suffer more serious consequences, including retarded growth and development [11,12], poor cognitive function

## Carcinoid syndrome

*Carcinoid symptoms are vasodilatory: flushing, diarrhea, palipitation.*

Refractory carcinoid syndrome: a review of treatment options - Rachel P. Riechelmann, Allan A. Pereira, Juliana F. M. Rego, Frederico P. Costa, 2017 (sagepub.com)

CSy is defined as symptoms and signs of overproduction of serotonin produced by neuroendocrine tumor, such as flushing, diarrhea, dyspnea, bronchospasm, palpitation, and eventually, symptoms associated with right-sided heart failure resulting from carcinoid heart [Bhattacharyya et al. 2007].

## Microscopic colitis

*Microscopic colitis is just general diarrhea, but it occurs way more often in older women.*

Sci-Hub | Diagnosis and Management of Microscopic Colitis | 10.1038/ajg.2016.477 (scihubtw.tw)

 The most common symptom in patients with microscopic colitis (MC) is chronic or intermittent watery diarrhea, ranging in severity from mild to severe with dehydration and electrolyte abnormalities. Other symptoms are commonly present, including abdominal pain, weight loss, and arthralgias, each present in up to half of patients

However, the presence or absence of certain clinical features, such as older age, female sex, use of certain medications or recent initiation of any medication, weight loss, nocturnal stools, and shorter duration of diarrhea, may identify patients at higher or lower risk of having MC

## Small intestinal bacterial overgrowth

*SIBO is mostly bloating or gas. PPIs are a big contributing factor.*

Small Intestinal Bacterial Overgrowth: Clinical Features and Therapeutic Management (nih.gov)

Although abdominal bloating, gas, distension, and diarrhea are common symptoms, they do not predict positive diagnosis. Predisposing factors include proton-pump inhibitors, opioids, gastric bypass, colectomy, and dysmotility.

**Eosinophilic gastroenteritis**

*Eosinophilic gastroenteritis is just diarrhea.*

Eosinophilic gastroenteritis: diagnosis and clinical perspectives (nih.gov)

Mucosal EGE is the most common variety, seen in about 57%7 to 100% of cases, and presents with features of abdominal pain, nausea, vomiting, dyspepsia, diarrhea, malabsorption, or protein-losing enteropathy, which in turn may cause hypoalbuminemia, anemia, and weight loss. Additionally, the occurrence of lower-GI bleeding may imply colonic involvement.

**Celiac disease**

*Celiac has some symptoms associated with it but nothing super indicative.*

Celiac disease: From pathophysiology to treatment (nih.gov)

Dermatitis herpetiformis is an inflammatory cutaneous disease, presenting with diffuse, symmetrical, polymorphic lesions consisting of erythema, urticarial plaques, papules, herpetiform vesiculae and blisters followed by erosions, excoriations and hyperpigmentation. It is characterized by typical histopathological and immunopathological findings. Rarely it is diagnosed in childhood but commonly appears in the third decade.

Type 1-diabetes

One of the most recognized and widely investigated disorders associated with celiac disease is type 1-diabetes

Autoimmune thyroid disorders

In patients affected by celiac disease it has been reported an increased prevalence (nearly, 2%-5%) of thyroid disorders (*i.e.*, hyperthyroidism-Graves's disease or hypothyroidism-Hashimoto's thyroiditis), diagnosed either before than after the diagnosis of gluten-enteropathy

Autoimmune hepatitis and other forms of liver involvement

The involvement of liver is common among patients affected by celiac disease

Life-long gluten-free diet

The current available treatment for celiac disease is life-long gluten-free diet[91-93]. Generally clinical improvement is achieved within a few weeks and the mucosal damage recovers in 1-2 years

**Bile acid malabsorption**

*Bile acid malabsorption is very hard to diagnose.*

Altered concentrations of bile acid (BA) in the colon can cause diarrhea or constipation. More than 25% of patients with irritable bowel syndrome with diarrhea or chronic diarrhea in Western countries have BA malabsorption (BAM)

Although BAM is recognized in practice, the most popular current method of diagnosis includes a therapeutic trial of BA binders with symptom improvement; this approach is prevalent and the only resource available in countries like the United States where the noninvasive imaging based on scintigraphic BA retention is unavailable. Unfortunately, in certain disease states, symptoms may only improve with high doses of a BA sequestrant or binder, and the diagnosis of BAM may be missed

## Dyssynergic defecation

*Dyssynergic defecation is mostly among older women.*

Diagnosis and Treatment of Dyssynergic Defecation (nih.gov)

Constipation is more common in women with an estimated female:male ratio of 2.2:1.[10] Its prevalence increases with advancing age, particularly after age 65.[10] African Americans,[10] lower socioeconomic status,[10] pregnancy,[14] and neurological diseases including Parkinson's disease and multiple sclerosis.

The etiology of dyssynergic defecation is unclear. In a prospective survey of 118 patients with dyssynergia, we found that the problem began during childhood in 31% of patients, and after a particular event, such as pregnancy, trauma, or back injury in 29% of patients, and there was no cause in 40% of patients

## Lactose intolerance

*Lactose intolerance is easiest to diagnose with lactose.*

Lactose Intolerance - American Family Physician (aafp.org)

Common symptoms include abdominal pain and bloating, excessive flatus, and watery stool following the ingestion of foods containing lactose. Lactase deficiency is present in up to 15 percent of persons of northern European descent, up to 80 percent of blacks and Latinos, and up to 100 percent of American Indians and Asians

## Non celiac gluten sensitivity

*Really tough to diagnose without an elimination diet.*

Recent advances in understanding non-celiac gluten sensitivity (nih.gov)

 In addition to experiencing GI symptoms, patients with NCGS most often experience a complex of extra-intestinal symptoms, including a "foggy mind", which is described as an inability to concentrate, reduction of mnemonic capabilities, and lack of well-being as well as tiredness, headache, anxiety, numbness, joint/muscle pain, and skin rash/dermatitis

According to self-reported data, the prevalence rate of NCGS ranges between 0.5% and 13% in the general population 2– 5, and prevalence is higher in women 2, 3, teenagers, and patients in the third to fourth decade of life 2, 4.

**Helicobacter pylori**

*Most characteristic symptom is ulcers.*

[A review of Helicobacter pylori diagnosis, treatment, and methods to detect eradication (nih.gov)](#)

*H. pylori* infection affects nearly half of the world's population. In developing countries, the prevalence of infection is as high as 90%, whereas in developed countries, excluding Japan, the prevalence is below 40%

Today, the involvement of H. pylori in active chronic gastritis, its association with gastroduodenal ulcer, and its well-accepted role as a risk factor for the development of gastric cancer are well documented[68].

[Gastritis | Cedars-Sinai (cedars-sinai.org)](#)

Stomach upset or pain

Belching and hiccups

Belly (abdominal) bleeding

Nausea and vomiting

Feeling of fullness or burning in your stomach

Loss of appetite

Blood in your vomit or stool. This is a sign that your stomach lining may be bleeding.


**Pelvic floor dysfunction**
*Variety of symptoms for pelvic floor dysfunction.*
[Sci-Hub | Recognition and Management of Nonrelaxing Pelvic Floor Dysfunction | 10.1016/j.mayocp.2011.09.004 (scihubtw.tw)](#)
Epidemiology
Women
Voluntarily hold urine or stool for long periods of time
Injury to pelvic floor from surgery, trauma, or long-term damage (i.e. bad posture)


Symptoms:

Bowel function: bloating, constipation, difficulty evacuating stool, straining with bowel movement, splinting the posterior vagina, anal digitation, incomplete evacuation, sense of anal blockage during defecation
Urinary function: frequency, hesitancy, urgency, dysuria, bladder pain, urge incontinence
Sexual function: insertional or deep dyspareunia, pelvic ache after intercourse
Pain: low back pain radiating to thighs or groin, pelvic pain unrelated to intercourse, lower abdominal wall pain

Note
Your doctor will need to perform a vaginal or rectal exam to fully diagnose

Treatment
Physical therapy

**Slow-transit constipation**
*Poor response to laxatives is the biggest indicator for slow-transit/colonic inertia.*
Thieme E-Journals - Clinics in Colon and Rectal Surgery / Abstract (thieme-connect.com)
Epidemiology
Old age, female gender, psychiatric illness, and history of sexual abuse

Symptoms
Constipation with straining
Poor response to laxatives

Note
Your doctor will need to perform a vaginal or rectal exam to fully diagnose

Treatment
Usually surgery

**Chronic idiopathic constipation**
*Not well defined from IBS-C.*
Sci-Hub | Prevalence of, and Risk Factors for, Chronic Idiopathic Constipation in the Community: Systematic Review and Meta-analysis | 10.1038/ajg.2011.164 (scihubtw.tw)
Epidemiology
Women, elderly, low socioeconomic status

Symptoms
Constipation
Straining
No physical abnormalities

Treatment

Same treatments as IBS

**General gastroparesis**
*Early satiety is the biggest tipoff.*

<u>Epidemiology</u>
Obesity
Diabetes

<u>Symptoms</u>
Early satiety
Nausea
Vomiting
Constipation

<u>Treatment</u>
Small meals
Lots of water
Low fiber
Some pharmaceuticals
Botox
Surgery

**Hirschprung's disease**
*Severe constipation since childhood is the biggest tipoff.*

<u>Epidemiology</u>

<u>Symptoms</u>
Severe constipation since childhood

<u>Treatment</u>
Surgery

**Diabetes**
*Diabetes is tough, because there aren't consistent symptoms. Obesity and pregnancy are tip offs for type II and gestational, while thirst and urination is a tipoff for type I.*
<u>Epidemiology</u>
Obesity (for type II)
Pregnancy (for gestational)

<u>Symptoms</u>
Weight loss (for type I)
Thirst (for type I)

Constipation

<u>Treatment</u>
Insulin
Dietary

**Uremia**
*This is really only a concern for people undergoing dialysis.*
<u>Epidemiology</u>
People undergoing dialysis
People with kidney problems

<u>Symptoms</u>
Anorexia
Lethargy

<u>Treatment</u>
Dialysis
Kidney transplant

**Parkinson's disease**
*Parkinson's tends to only be noticed once it gets to the characteristic motor symptoms.*
<u>Epidemiology</u>
People over the age of 65
People who were exposed to chemicals or herbicides in their youth

<u>Symptoms</u>
Shuffling walk
Tremor
Loss of smell
Sleep disturbance

<u>Treatment</u>
Prescription medication (dopamine agonists)

**Multiple sclerosis**
*Optical neuritis is the most characteristic symptom of MS.*
<u>Epidemiology</u>
Women
Age 20-40 years

<u>Symptoms</u>
Pain or loss of vision in one eye over hours or days
Sharp shooting pain down legs or arms

Increased sensitivity to cold, touch, or heat
Numbness or tingling
Blurred or double vision
Muscle weakness

<u>Treatment</u>
Prescription medication

## A note on sources

If it's not sourced, I probably got it from Wikipedia. God bless that website.


## If you want updates to this book

I'll be updating this book periodically with studies, papers, and information on IBS and related disorders. If you're interested, sign up for the newsletter: https://landing.mailerlite.com/webforms/landing/k8d5n9 .